Notes on Medical Virology

Morag C. Timbury

MD, PhD, FRSE, FRCP (Glasg.), FRC Path

Professor and William Teacher Lecturer in Bacteriology,
University of Glasgow, Honorary Consultant Virologist,
Royal Infirmary and Regional Virus Laboratory,
Ruchill Hospital, Glasgow, UK

FOREWORD BY

J.H. Subak-Sharpe

BSc, PhD, FRSE

Professor of Virology, University of Glasgow, Glasgow, UK

EIGHTH EDITION

CHURCHILL LIVINGSTONE
EDINBURGH LONDON MELBOURNE AND NEW YORK 1986

CHURCHILL LIVINGSTONE
Medical Division of Longman Group UK Limited

Distributed in the United States of America by
Churchill Livingstone Inc., 1560 Broadway, New
York, N.Y. 10036, and by associated companies,
branches and representatives throughout the world.

First edition 1967
Second edition 1969
Third edition 1971
Fourth edition 1973
Fifth edition 1974
Sixth edition 1978
Seventh edition 1983
Eighth edition 1986
  Reprinted 1987
  Reprinted 1988

ISBN 0-443-03328-5

British Library Cataloguing in Publication Data
Timbury, Morag C.
    Notes on medical virology.—8th eld.—
    (Churchill Livingstone medical text)
    1. Viruses.   2. Micro-organisms, Pathogenic
    I. Title
    616'.0194   QR360

Library of Congress Cataloging in Publication Data
Timbury, Morag Crichton.
    Notes on medical virology.

    (Churchill Livingstone medical text)
    Based on the lecture course given to medical students
    at the University of Glasgow.
    Bibliography: p.
    Includes index.
    1. Virus diseases.   I. Title.   II. Series
[DNLM: 1. Virus Diseases. 2. Viruses. WC 500 T583n]
RC114.5.T55   1986   616',0194   85-16672

Produced by Longman Singapore Publishers (Pte) Ltd.
Printed in Singapore.

Notes on Medical Virology

CHURCHILL LIVINGSTONE MEDICAL TEXTS

Foreword

Virology concerns itself with viruses at many different levels — from the study at the molecular level of the structure, genetic information, content and function of the particle and the virus-host cell complex, via the analysis of the events which define the progress of viral disease in the host organism to interrelationships between the virus and populations of potential host organisms. These different levels necessarily have led to a dichotomy of virology into the pure and the applied field and, until now, medicine for all practical purposes has been almost solely concerned with the latter. But, as our knowledge of viruses at all analytical levels is becoming more and more extensive, and particularly if one considers the recent dramatic increase of our understanding of events at the molecular level, some knowledge of the general field of pure virology is bound to become relevant even for the doctor in general practice whose sole concern in the past has been with the field of applied virology. These notes are starting to bridge this gap.

Professor Timbury's lucid, concise and astonishingly comprehensive book of notes is particularly well suited to help medical students, who are primarily concerned with the spectrum of diseases caused by viruses, to get acquainted with the subject of virology. The book neither aims nor pretends to be a self-sufficient textbook, and, to this end, recommended books for further reading have been included. Clearly presented, informative and inexpensive, this book should prove most useful to students in conjunction with their course of lectures, practicals and hospital instruction.

The book, which is an excellent summary of the major virological problems in medicine, can be highly recommended for students of medicine.

J.H. Subak-Sharpe

Preface

This book originated from lecture notes which were handed out to accompany my virology lectures to the medical students in Glasgow University. I wrote it in the same concise note form to try and present clearly the facts about virus diseases which students have to know for their professional examination in microbiology. Although it is meant to be reasonably comprehensive, students should refer to some of the larger books on the subject and I have listed some of my favourites on page 152.

Many colleagues have helped me with advice and discussion on numerous points, notably Professor C.R. Pringle, University of Warwick, to whom I am particularly grateful. Thanks are also due to Dr Follett, Dr Helen Laird and Professor Madeley for the photographs and to Mr R. Callander for the drawings and diagrams.

Finally, I should like to thank Professor J.H. Subak-Sharpe, not only for the Foreword but for the many happy years I spent in his department, and Professor N.R. Grist in whose laboratory I first acquired my interest in viruses.

Glasgow 1986   M.C.T.

Contents

1

General properties of viruses

Viruses are the smallest known infective agents. Most forms of life—animals, plants and bacteria—are susceptible to infection with appropriate viruses.

Three main properties distinguish viruses from other micro-organisms:

1. *Small size*. Viruses are smaller than other organisms and vary in size from 10 nm to 300 nm. In contrast, bacteria are approximately 1000 nm and erythrocytes are 7500 nm in diameter.
2. *Genome*. The genome of viruses may be either DNA or RNA; viruses contain only one type of nucleic acid.
3. *Metabolically inert*. Viruses have no metabolic activity outside susceptible host cells; they do not possess any ribosomes or protein-synthesising apparatus although some viruses contain enzymes within their particles; viruses cannot therefore multiply in inanimate media but only inside living cells. On entry into a susceptible cell, however, the virus genome or nucleic acid is transcribed into—or itself acts as—virus-specific messenger or mRNA which then directs the replication of new virus particles.

STRUCTURE OF VIRUSES

Viruses consist basically of a core of nucleic acid surrounded by a protein coat.

The protein coat protects the viral genome from inactivation by adverse environmental factors, e.g. nucleases in the blood stream. It is antigenic and often responsible for stimulating the production of protective antibodies.

The structures which make up a virus particle are known as:

Virion—the intact virus particle.

Capsid—the protein coat.

1

Capsomeres—the protein structural units of which the capsid is composed.

Nucleic acid

Envelope: the particles of many viruses are surrounded by a lipo-protein envelope containing viral antigens but also partially derived from the outer membrane of the host cell.

Virus particles show three types of symmetry:

Cubic—in which the particles are icosahedral protein shells with the nucleic acid contained inside (Fig. 1.1).

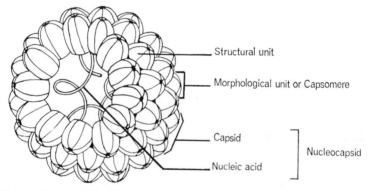

Fig. 1.1 Diagram of icosahedral virus particle with cubic symmetry. (Reproduced, with permission, from *Virus Morphology* by C.R. Madeley.)

Helical—in which the particle is elongated and wound in the form of a helix or spiral; the capsomeres are arranged round the spiral of nucleic acid. Most helical viruses possess an outer envelope (Fig. 1.2).

Complex—in which the particle does not confirm to either cubic or helical symmetry.

CULTIVATION OF VIRUSES

Since viruses will only replicate within living cells special methods have to be employed for culture *in vitro*; three main systems are used for their cultivation in the laboratory (see Chapter 3).

1. *Tissue culture*. Cells obtained from man or animals are grown in artificial culture in glass vessels in the laboratory; these cells are living and metabolising and so can support viral replication. Most viruses can be propagated in cultures of suitable cells.

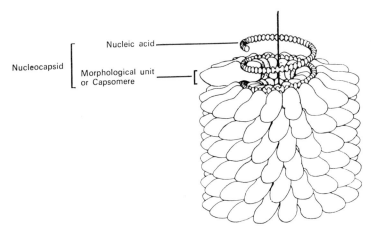

Fig. 1.2 Diagram of nucleocapsid of virus particle with helical symmetry. (Reproduced, with permission, from *Advances in Virus Research*, 1960, p. 274)

2. *Chick embryo.* Some viruses grow in the cells of the chick embryo; fertile eggs are kept in an incubator in the laboratory for this purpose. This technique has been largely superseded by tissue culture.

2. *Laboratory animals.* Before other techniques were available, viruses were isolated and studied mainly by inoculation of laboratory animals such as mice, rabbits, ferrets and monkeys; animals are still required for the isolation of a few viruses.

EFFECTS OF VIRUSES ON CELLS

Viruses may affect cells in three ways:

Cell death. The infection is lethal and kills the cell causing a cytopathic effect (CPE).

Cell transformation. The cell is not killed but is changed from a normal cell to one with the properties of a malignant or cancerous cell.

Latent infection. The virus remains within the cell in a potentially active state but produces no obvious effect on the cell's functions.

Haemadsorption

Some viruses have protein (haemagglutinin) in their outer coats which adheres to erythrocytes causing them to agglutinate: in tissue culture, these viruses produce haemagglutinin on the surface of infected cells to which added erythrocytes adhere.

Table 1.1 Virus classification and diseases

Family	Viruses	Diseases
DNA viruses		
Poxviruses	Variola, molluscum	Smallpox, molluscum contagiosum
Herpesviruses	Herpes simplex, varicella-zoster, cytomegalovirus, EB virus	Herpes, chickenpox, shingles, infectious mononucleosis
Adenoviruses	Adenoviruses	Sore throats, conjunctivitis
Papovaviruses	Papilloma, polyoma, SV_{40}	Warts, progressive multifocal leucoencephalopathy
Parvoviruses	Parvovirus	Erythema infectiosum haemolytic crises
RNA viruses		
Orthomyxoviruses	Influenza	Influenza
Paramyxoviruses	Parainfluenza, respiratory syncytial, measles, mumps,	Respiratory, measles, mumps
Rhabdoviruses	Rabies	Rabies
Picornaviruses	Enteroviruses, rhinoviruses	Meningitis, poliomyelitis, colds
Togaviruses	Alphaviruses, flaviviruses	Encephalitis, febrile disease
Reoviruses	Rotavirus	Infantile diarrhoea
Arenaviruses	Lymphocytic choriomeningitis, Lassa virus	Meningitis, febrile disease
Retroviruses	HTLV I, II, III	T-cell leukaemia-lymphoma AIDS

CLASSIFICATION

Viruses are assigned to groups mainly on the basis of the morphology of the virus particle, but also of their nucleic acid and method of RNA transcription.

The main groups of medically-important viruses and the morphology of their particles are shown in Table 1.1.

THE EFFECT OF PHYSICAL AND CHEMICAL AGENTS ON VIRUSES

Heat. Most are inactivated at 56°C for 30 minutes or at 100°C for a few seconds.

Cold. Stable at low temperatures, most can be stored at −40°C or, preferably, at −70°C; some viruses are partially inactivated by the process of freezing and thawing.

Drying. Variable. Some survive well, others are rapidly inactivated.

Ultra-violet irradiation. Inactivates viruses.

Chloroform and ether. Viruses with lipid-containing envelopes are inactivated, those without envelopes are resistant.

Oxidising and reducing agents. Viruses are inactivated by formaldehyde, chlorine, iodine and hydrogen peroxide.

Phenols. Most viruses are relatively resistant.

Virus disinfectants. The best are hypochlorite solution (which is corrosive) and gluteraldehyde.

VIRUS DISEASES

Viruses are important and common causes of human disease, especially in children. Most viral infections are mild and the patient makes a complete recovery; many infections are silent and the virus multiples in the body without causing symptoms of disease.

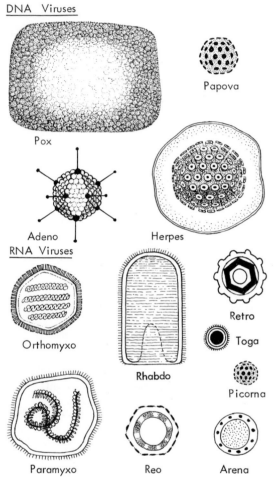

Fig. 1.3 Diagram showing the structure of the particles of different families of virus.

However, viral infections which are usually mild may occasionally cause severe disease in an unusually susceptible patient; a few viral diseases are severe and always have a high mortality rate.

Entry

Viruses most often enter the body via the respiratory tract by inhalation but some viruses gain entry by ingestion, by inoculation through skin abrasions or via the bite of an arthropod vector.

Virus diseases can be of two types:

1. *Systemic*. The virus spreads widely and invades many tissues and organs as a result of viraemia or virus in the blood stream; there is a relatively long incubation period, e.g. childhood fevers such as measles and varicella.

2. *Localized*. The virus invades only tissues adjacent to the site of entry; the incubation period is usually short. Most respiratory virus infections are of this type.

Invasiveness

Virus disease is produced by direct spread of the virus to tissues and organs and not to toxin production as in bacteria. The process of virus replication in the cells of the tissues usually—but not always—kills the infected cells; this may result in lesions and disease in the tissue concerned.

HOST RESPONSE TO VIRUS INFECTION

The body defences are of two types:

1. Non-specific
2. Specific

Non-specific defence mechanisms

1. *Interferon*: probably the principal mechanism by which the body overcomes acute virus infection: interferon is a complex of protein regulatory molecules which are released from virus-infected cells; when taken up by uninfected cells these are rendered resistant to virus infection: interferon is demonstrable in blood and tissues during the acute phase of virus infections: it is host cell specific but acts against all viruses. It is of low toxicity and can be prepared (but only in small quantities) *in vitro*: it is therefore a promising anti-viral agent (see Chap. 14).

2. *Phagocytosis*: a most important defence mechanism in bacterial infection and probably in virus infections also: invading viruses—like bacteria—are ingested by two types of scavenger cell:

   (i) Neutrophil polymorphonuclear leucocytes
   (ii) Macrophages (or mononuclear cells of the reticuloendothelial system):
   a. free macrophages in lung alveoli, peritoneum

    b. fixed macrophages in lymph nodes, spleen, liver (Kupffer cells), connective tissue (histiocytes) and CNS (microglia)

    Phagocytosis is enhanced by antibody (which is, of course, a specific mechanism) and complement: this effect is known as *opsonization*.

3. *Respiratory tract*: the constant upward movement due to the action of ciliated epithelium and the 'washing' effect of mucus
4. *Stomach acid*: inactivates acid-labile viruses
5. *Skin*: forms an impermeable barrier unless breached by injury, infection etc.

Specific defence mechanisms

Specific mechanisms are due to the immune system:
they are specific in that they react only with the virus which elicited their production: the immune system has two main components:

1. Humoral immunity (due to antibody)
2. Cell-mediate immunity due to lymphocytes

1. Humoral immunity

Antibodies are immunoglobulins, i.e. proteins which react specifically with antigens (also usually proteins) in virus particles: produced by plasma cells formed when B-lymphocytes become activated after encountering antigen in spleen or lymphocytes: T-lymphocytes act as helper cells in the initial interaction between antigen and B-lymphocytes.

    Antiviral action: virus antibodies *neutralize* virus infectivity i.e. they render viruses non-infectious: this is an extremely effective mechanism and is responsible for the long-term immunity which usually follows virus infection.

    Immunoglobulins have a Y-shaped structure: the stem is the Fc fragment: the two arms are the Fab fragments and contain the antibody-combining sites: there are three main immunoglobulins which are responsible for the immune response in virus infection:

(i) *IgM*: the earliest antibody produced: formed about a week after infection, it persists for about 4–6 weeks: a pentamer of five IgG molecules.

(ii) *IgG*: formed later than IgM but persists for months and often years: responsible for the immunity to reinfection.

(iii) *IgA*: a dimeric molecule: found in body secretions as well as blood, e.g. saliva, respiratory secretions, tears and intestinal contents: acquired a carbohydrate 'transport piece' in extracellular fluids but this is absent in serum IgA: the main antibody responsible for immunity to respiratory viruses and for the gut immunity seen after enterovirus infection.

2. Cell-mediated immunity

This, the delayed hypersensitivity response, acts to limit or localise the lesions of virus infections.

T-(or thymus-dependent) lymphocytes: are the main cells involved: when sensitised or primed, T-lymphocytes react specifically with antigen and transform into blast cells with release of lymphokines.

Lymphokines attract by chemotaxis, lymphocytes, macrophages and polymorphonuclear leucocytes to the site of infection.

Other factors which influence virus infection

Age

Virus infections are generally acquired in childhood and are followed by long-lasting, sometimes lifelong, immunity: a few infections of the recurrent type are more common in the elderly.

Immune deficiency

In which the host's defence mechanisms are impaired: generally results in increased susceptibility to infection: may be due to:
a. Therapy: immunosuppressive, cytotoxic drugs or radiotherapy.
b. Disease: AIDS, malignancy (especially leukaemia or lymphoma): some other chronic debilitating diseases: rarely, congenital immune deficiency especially that affecting cell-mediated immunity (e.g. Di George's syndrome, Swiss type hypogammaglobulinaemia).
c. Transplantation: involves deliberate immunosuppression, and impairs the host response to virus infection.

Pregnancy

Certain viruses are able to cross the placental barrier to invade the fetus: this may cause congenital abnormalities or—usually severe—infection of the fetus.

2

Virus replication

Viruses have no metabolic activity of their own: they replicate by taking over the biochemical machinery of the host cell and redirecting it to the manufacture of virus components. This take-over is achieved by *virus mRNA*.

VIRUS GROWTH CYCLE

Takes place in seven stages:
1. **Adsorption**
    (i) to specific receptors on the cell plasma membrane
    (ii) best at 37°C but also—although slowly—at 4°C
    (iii) enhanced by Mg^{++} or Ca^{++}.
2. **Entry**
    (i) complex: probably by invagination of cell membrane round virus particle to enclose it in a pinocytotic vacuole
    (ii) with syncytia-producing viruses by fusion of virus envelope with cell membrane.
3. **Uncoating**
    (i) releases—or renders accessible—the virus nucleic acid or genome
    (ii) cell enzymes (from lysosomes) strip off the virus protein coat.
4. **Transcription**
    (i) the production of virus mRNA or replicative intermediates from the viral genome
    (ii) carried out by either host cell or virus-specified enzyme
    (iii) subject to complex control mechanisms:
        a. patterns of transcription may differ before (early) and after (late) virus nucleic acid replication
        b. primary transcripts are often spliced to remove intron sequences between expressed exons

c. transcription is sometimes overlapping with different starting and/or termination points within one gene to produce different proteins from the same nucleic acid sequence.

Virus mRNA generally, but not invariably:
i. contains leader sequences
ii. capped at the 5' end
iii. polyadenylated at the 3' terminus.

5. **Synthesis of virus components**

Virus protein synthesis:
(i) virus mRNA is translated on cell ribosomes
(ii) into two types of virus protein:
  a. structural—the proteins which make up the virus particle
  b. non-structural—not found in the particle, mainly enzymes for virus genome replication

Virus nucleic acid synthesis:
(i) new virus genomes are synthesized
(ii) templates are either the parental genome or, with single-stranded nucleic acid genomes, newly formed complementary strands
(iii) most often by a virus-coded polymerase or replicase: with some DNA viruses a cell enzyme carries this out.

6. **Assembly**
(i) new virus genomes and proteins come together to form new virus particles
(ii) may take place in cell nucleus, cytoplasm or (with most enveloped viruses) at the plasma membrane which invests the new particle to form the virus envelope.

7. **Release**
(i) either by sudden rupture or by gradual extrusion (budding) of enveloped viruses through the cell membranes.

VIRUS GENOMES

Nucleic acid

(i) may be DNA or RNA
(ii) single or double-stranded
(iii) intact or fragmented, linear or circular
(iv) some viruses (adeno and polio) have a small protein covalently bonded to the 5' terminus.

Large viruses

(i) have high molecular weight nucleic acid
(ii) can code for many proteins
(iii) code for many of the enzymes involved in replication

Small viruses

(i) have low molecular weight nucleic acid

Table 2.1 Some properties of viruses and their genomes

| Virus family | Example | Type[a] | Nucleic acid | | Transcriptase contained in virus particles |
			Molecular weight ($\times 10^6$)	Infectivity	
Pox	Vaccinia	DS DNA	160	0	+
Herpes	Herpes simplex	DS DNA	100	+	0
Adeno	Adenovirus	DS DNA	23	+	0
Papova	Polyoma	DS DNA	3	+	0
Parvo	Parvovirus H1	SS DNA	1.7	+	0
Picorna	Poliovirus	SS RNA	2.6	+	0
Calici	Feline calicivirus	SS RNA	2.7	+	0
Toga	Sindbis	SS RNA	4.0	+	0
Corona	Murine hepatitis	SS RNA	5.8	+	0
Orthomyxo	Influenza A	SS RNA[c]	5.7	0	+
Arena	Lassa fever	SS RNA[c]	3.2	0	+
Bunya	Crimean haemorrhagic fever	SS RNA[c]	6.4	0	+
Rhabdo	Rabies	SS RNA	4	0	+
Paramyxo	Parainfluenza	SS RNA	7.0	0	+
Retro	Rous sarcoma	SS RNA[d]	3.0	0[e]	+[b]
Diplornavirus	Rotavirus	DS RNA[c]	11	0	+

a DS = double-stranded; SS = single stranded
b reverse transcriptase
c fragmented (diplorna 10–12 unique sub-units, orthomyxo 7–8, bunya 3, arena 2)
d two identical sub-units in the virion
e provirus infectious

(ii) therefore limited coding capacity

(iii) must use some of the cell enzymes for replication

Infectivity

(i) with many viruses the purified nucleic acid genome is infectious when applied to cells—i.e. without the capsid, nucleic acid on its own can infect a cell to initiate a complete infectious cycle of virus replication.

(ii) virus genomes of which the virions contain a transcriptase, are non-infectious: this is because the process of nucleic acid extraction removes the virion transciptase and mRNA cannot then be produced.

The properties of the main virus groups and their genomes are shown in Table 2.1.

Baltimore classification

This classifies viruses into six groups on the basis of their nucleic acid and mRNA production (Fig. 2.1).

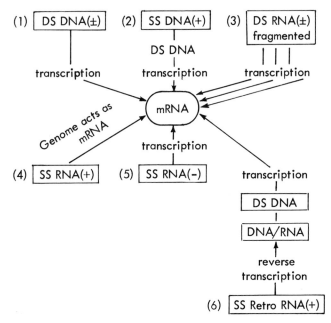

Fig. 2.1 Diagram to show methods of transcription of the six different groups in the Baltimore classification of virus genomes

BIOCHEMISTRY OF VIRUS REPLICATION

An extremely complex subject: a few examples only will be outlined here to highlight the main differences in the growth cycles of some respresentative groups of viruses.

Double-stranded DNA viruses

Examples: vaccinia, herpes simplex, adeno, polyoma viruses. The principal steps in their growth cycle are detailed below and shown diagrammatically in Fig. 2.2.

Transcription: two main types of mRNAs are produced:
1. *Early* mRNA—before virus DNA synthesis—codes mainly for enzymes and for control proteins
2. *Late* mRNA—after virus DNA synthesis—codes mainly for structural proteins.

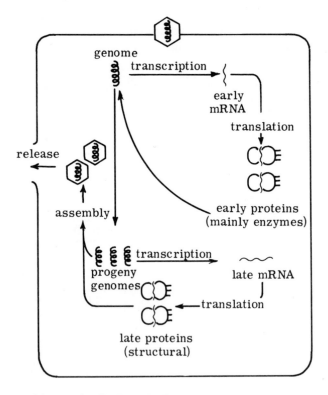

Fig. 2.2 Diagram of replicative cycle of double-stranded DNA virus.

Virus DNA synthesis:
Enzymes: many are involved but
1. the main DNA replicative enzyme is DNA-dependent DNA polymerase
2. larger viruses code for their own enzyme (vaccinia, herpes simplex)
3. smaller viruses use the host cell DNA polymerase (adeno, polyoma)

Template: new progeny virus DNA is synthesised off the DNA genome of the input parental virus.

Site: nucleus (except pox viruses)

New progeny DNA: acts as templates for:
1. transcription of late virus mRNA
2. synthesis of more genomes for new virus particles.

Virus protein synthesis: is a two-stage process:
1. production of early proteins required for
    (i) virus DNA synthesis (e.g. DNA-dependent DNA polymerase, thymidine kinase, other enzymes)
    (ii) control of transcription
2. production of late proteins
    (i) produced after virus DNA synthesis
    (ii) mostly the capsid proteins for new particles.

Site: virus proteins are synthesized on the ribosomes in the cell cytoplasm and then transported to sites of assembly.

Assembly: of new DNA genomes and proteins into new infectious particles within the cell takes place in:
1. *Nucleus*—herpes simplex, adeno, polyoma viruses:
    Note: herpes particles acquire an envelope by budding through the cell nuclear membrane which has been modified by the incorporation within it of virus glycoproteins.
2. *Cytoplasm*—vaccinia replicates entirely in the cytoplasm in "factories" which are based on clusters of ribosomes.

Other DNA viruses

Hepatitis B virus is at present unclassified: it has the smallest known

DNA genome (3150 base pairs compared with the 5310 of polyoma virus). The infectious particle contains an incompletely double-stranded DNA molecule of 1.6×10^6 mol. wt. and a DNA polymerase which can fill in the gap to produce a completely double-stranded molecule of 2.1×10^6 mol. wt. The genes for the surface and core proteins overlap (and presumably so too does the gene for the DNA polymerase). Replication of the genome is unique in that it appears to involve a negative-strand RNA template generated by reverse transcription to produce a RNA/DNA intermediate which is subsequently converted to double-stranded DNA.

Parvoviruses: have a tiny single-stranded DNA genome. Some are *autonomous* in replication (eg. human parvovirus), others are *defective* and require a helper virus for replication (e.g. adeno-associated virus which is dependent on a helper adenovirus). Autonomous parvoviruses generally package within their virions only minus or negative strand DNA (i.e. strands from which virus mRNA is transcribed): defective viruses package both plus and minus strand DNA but separately within different particles. Both autonomous and defective viruses have terminally redundant DNA but in the former the repeated regions are different whereas with the defective viruses they have identical sequences. The parvovirus genome codes for three structural proteins from overlapping sequences.

RNA viruses

Because their genetic material is RNA, these viruses use biochemical mechanisms for their replication which are different from those of other forms of living organisms.

RNA virus genomes have different methods of transcription:

1. *Single plus strand RNA*: the virus genome is the virus mRNA
2. *Single negative strand RNA*: virus mRNA is transcribed from the parental genome
3. *Double stranded fragmented RNA*: individual virus mRNAs are transcribed separately off the parental RNA segments using a transcriptase associated with each segment
4. *Retrovirus*: the virus genome alternates between RNA and DNA: parental single-stranded RNA is transcribed into double-stranded DNA and integrated into the host genome as a "provirus" from which virus RNA is later transcribed.

Below are selected examples of the replication cycle of some RNA viruses.

Single plus strand RNA viruses

Example: poliovirus.

With these viruses, there is no transcription stage because the single plus strand RNA genome acts itself as virus mRNA. The replication cycle is shown diagrammatically in Fig. 2.3.

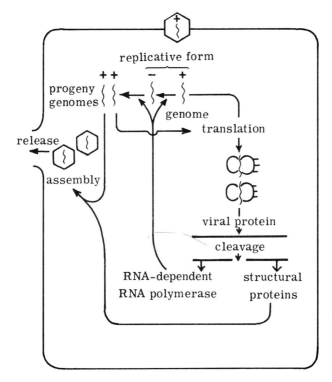

Fig. 2.3 Diagram of replicative cycle of plus strand RNA virus

Translation

The virus genome is translated into one very large polypeptide which is almost immediately cleaved into smaller proteins as follows:

1. structural viral capsid proteins
2. the RNA-dependent RNA polymerase required for replication of virus RNA (no similar enzyme exists in cells)
3. a protease for processing the precursor polypeptide, and the genome-linked terminal protein.

Virus RNA synthesis

New genome production takes place on a double-stranded 'replicative form' made by the synthesis of a negative RNA strand complementary to the input plus-stranded parental RNA.

New progeny plus strands are synthesized off the template of the negative RNA strand in the replicative form.

RNA-dependent RNA polymerase synthesizes both the replicative form and also new plus-strand genomes.

Progeny (plus) strand RNA functions as:
1. templates for the production of more replicative forms (and so for more genome RNA synthesis)
2. genomes for new virus particles
3. virus mRNA.

Assembly

New progeny virus particles are assembled from the cleavage products of the primary translation product and from progeny virus RNA in the cytoplasm on clusters of ribosomes: poliovirus replicates entirely in the cytoplasm.

Release

By sudden rupture of the cell.

Single negative strand RNA viruses

Example: parainfluenza virus.
The replicative cycle is shown diagrammatically in Fig. 2.4.

Transcription

Virus mRNA is synthesized off the parental (negative strand) genome RNA using a transcriptase (RNA-dependent RNA polymerase) contained in the virus particle.
    Separate virus mRNAs for the different proteins are formed either by:
1. control of transcription
2. processing of the primary transcript.

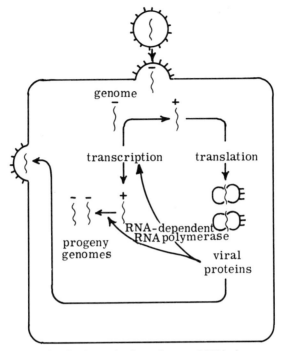

Fig. 2.4 Diagram of replicative cycle of negative strand RNA virus

Virus RNA synthesis

Virus progeny genomes are produced—also by the transcriptase—using RNA positive strands complementary to the parental genome as templates.

Virus protein synthesis

Virus proteins include
1. transcriptase
2. envelope proteins (two are glycosylated and have haemagglutinin/neuraminidase and fusion/haemolysis activities respectively)
3. nucleocapsid proteins.

Assembly

New virus nucleocapsids are assembled at the cell membrane and become enveloped by budding through the plasma membrane.

Note: *infuenza* virus has a fragmented genome each fragment of which codes for a different virus protein.

Double stranded RNA viruses

All double stranded RNA viruses have *fragmented genomes*. Each fragment codes for a different protein and each is associated with a molecule of transcriptase (RNA-dependent RNA polymerase). The replicative cycle starts with transcription of mRNA from each double-stranded RNA fragment—the mRNAs produced then being translated into the different virus proteins. These mRNA molecules later become enclosed within nucleocapsids together with a transcriptase which directs the synthesis of a complementary RNA strand to produce the double-stranded fragments which make up the genome.

Retrovirus

Example: Rous sarcoma virus.
Retroviruses are tumour viruses which can replicate in cells without killing them and may also *transform* normal cells into malignant or cancer cells. Their replication involves the production of virus DNA which integrates into the cell chromosome.

The retrovirus genome: is single-stranded dimeric RNA with four genes:

gag—core proteins

pol—polymerase—reverse transcriptase (contained in the virion)

env—envelope proteins

onc—(oncogene) transforming protein

In Rous sarcoma virus: the oncogene is known as *src* (sarcoma) gene and is a specific type of *onc* gene which produces a 60K molecular weight phosphoprotein. The virus *src* gene (v-*src*) is related to a normal host cell gene (c-*src*). Virus *onc* (i.e. v-*onc*) genes generally represent variants of specific host cell genes (c-*onc*) picked up by the virus as rare events in evolution.

The replicative cycle is shown diagrammatically in Fig. 2.5.
First stage: 1. *transcription* (by the reverse transcriptase contained

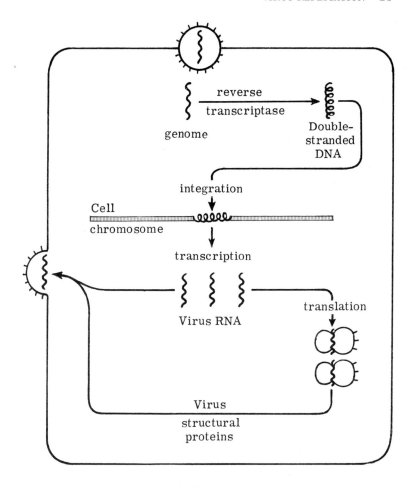

Fig. 2.5 Diagram of replicative cycle of retrovirus

in the virion) to produce a DNA/RNA genome heteroduplex.

2. *conversion* of the DNA/RNA heteroduplex into double-stranded DNA.

3. *integration* of the double-stranded virus DNA into the cellular chromosome where it is known as *provirus*.

Second stage: 1. provirus DNA is transcribed (by cell enzyme)

2. the RNA transcripts produced have two functions—

i. *mRNA* for translation into virus proteins
ii. *new virus genomes*

Virus protein synthesis: Virus proteins are produced on cell ribosomes by translation of mRNA transcribed off the provirus DNA.
1. reverse transcriptase
2. core proteins
3. envelope proteins
4. transforming protein

Assembly: virus nucleocapsides are assembled from the progeny virus RNA genomes and proteins at the cell surface and acquire their outer-envelope by budding through the cell plasma membrane.

3

Laboratory diagnosis of virus infection

Virus diseases are diagnosed by:
1. **Serology**, i.e. demonstration of virus antibody
2. **Isolation** of virus
3. **Direct demonstration** of virus or antigen in material from the patient.

SEROLOGY

By far the most widely used way to diagnose virus infection. Serological diagnosis depends on the detection of virus antibody.

Detection of virus antibody

Virus antibodies are common in healthy populations and can remain at a high level for many years after infection. A diagnosis of recent infection depends on the following criteria:
1. *Detection of IgM*: the earliest antibody to appear and therefore only present if there has been recent infection with the virus. IgM can be demonstrated by fractionating serum in a sucrose density gradient or by using anti-IgM antibody to detect it serologically.
2. *Rising titre*: i.e. increase in the level of virus antibody at least four-fold over the course of infection from the acute phase into convalescence. (**Note**: titre is the highest dilution of an antiserum at which activity is demonstrated: usually expressed as the reciprocal of the antiserum dilution, i.e. 64 rather than 1/64).
3. *High stationary titre*: unreliable: but if the titre of antibody is *considerably* higher than that found in the general population, recent infection with the virus can be assumed.

Tests used in serology

The old but well-tried and reliable technique of complement fixation test is now being replaced by more sensitive assays—especially those which detect virus-specific IgM.

Below are some of the most widely used tests:

1. **Immunofluorescence**: Virus-specific antibody is detected usually by the indirect or sandwich technique (Fig. 3.1). In this, dilutions of patient's serum are added to spots of virus-infected cells on microscope slides. After washing, virus antibody is detected on the cells by application of fluorescein-labelled anti-human IgG or IgM. Fluorescence is detected by examination in a microscope under ultra-violet light and indicates the presence of virus antibody and—according to the highest dilution of the patient's serum at which this is observed—the titre of antibody. Sometimes virus antibody is detected by addition of complement to the reaction and then detecting its fixation by fluorescein-labelled anti-complement antibody.

2. **Enzyme-linked immunoabsorbent assay (ELISA)**: Similar in principle to immunofluorescence but instead of fluorescein-labelled anti-human antibody to detect virus antibody, the label used is an enzyme which reacts with a suitable substrate to produce a visible colour change. The enzyme-substrates most often used are:

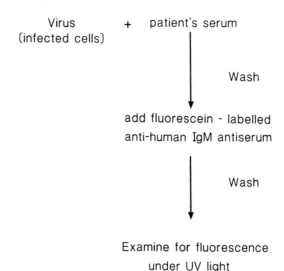

Fig. 3.1 Diagram of indirect immunofluorescent test for virus IgM antibody

    i. Horseradish peroxidase and hydrogen peroxide: ortho-phenyldiamine

    ii. Alkaline phosphatase: paranitrophenyl phosphate.

3. **Radio-immune assay (RIA)**: Generally the most sensitive technique. Also similar in principle to immunofluorescence but the detecting anti-human antibody is tagged with an isotope—most often I^{125}.

Antibody capture tests: Both ELISA and RIA tests can be made more sensitive and more specific by 'capturing' patient's IgM, reacting it with virus and then by adding labelled monoclonal antiviral antibody. This is illustrated in Fig. 3.2.

4. **Complement fixation test**: Virus antibody is detected by the fixation of added complement when the antibody combines with virus antigen. The fixation is rendered visible by later addition of 'sensitised' (i.e. by mixing with anti-erythrocyte antibody) sheep erythrocytes (Fig. 3.3). If virus antibody is present complement is fixed and the sheep red cells do not haemolyse: if no virus antibody is present the complement lyses the sensitized erythrocytes.

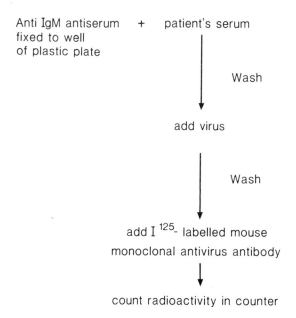

Fig. 3.2 Diagram of radio-immune assay (antibody capture test) for virus IgM antibody

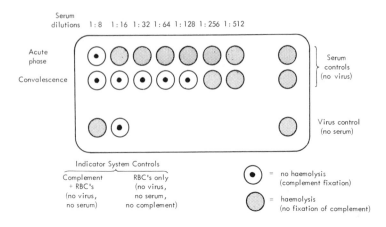

Fig. 3.3 Diagram of complement-fixation test for viral antibody. Virus antigen is mixed overnight at 4°C with dilutions of the patient's serum and complement before addition of sensitised sheep erythrocytes. Titre of complement-fixing antibody has risen from 8 in the acute phase to 128 in convalescence—a greater than 4-fold rise in titre indicating recent infection.

5. **Haemagglutination-inhibition test**: Many viruses haemagglutinate erythrocytes but virus antibody blocks this. Antibody can be detected in a patient's serum by inhibition of virus haemagglutination (Fig. 3.4).

6. **Radial immune haemolysis**: A useful qualitative test for antibody detection—but not titration—with haemagglutinating viruses. Virus, complement and erythrocytes are mixed in an agar gel in a plate. Patients' sera are added to wells cut in the agar: if antibody is present, zones of haemolysis appear round the wells on incubation.

7. **Neutralization**: Antibody prevents virus infection of cells. Antibody can be detected by neutralization of virus CPE in tissue culture.

VIRUS ISOLATION

Virus isolation requires the use of living cells since viruses cannot grow on inanimate media. There are three main systems:

1. Tissue culture
2. Chick embryo
3. Laboratory animals } now rarely used

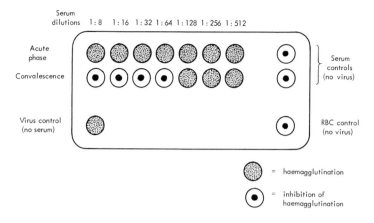

Fig. 3.4 Diagram of haemagglutination-inhibition test for viral antibody. The haemagglutinating virus is mixed with dilutions of the patient's serum for one hour before addition of erythrocytes. Titre of haemagglutination-inhibiting antibody has risen from less than 8 in the acute phase to 64 in convalescence—a greater than 4-fold rise in titre indicating recent infection.

1. Tissue culture

Tissue culture is really cell culture and consists of a single layer (monolayer) of actively metabolising cells adherent to a glass or plastic surface in a test tube, petri plate or on one side of a flat bottle.

The main types of tissue culture are:

1. *Primary cultures*: are laborious to prepare and short-lived but generally susceptible to a wide range of viruses. There is little cell division and although one subculture can be done, the cells die in about two to three weeks, e.g. monkey kidney and human amnion.

2. *Semi-continuous cell strains*: are established from human embryo lung: easy to maintain and can be subcultured for about 30 to 40 passages before the cells die off. Susceptible to a wide range of viruses.

3. *Continuous cell lines*: can be subcultured indefinitely and are therefore easy to maintain. Generally susceptible to fewer viruses than the other types of cell culture. HeLa (derived from human cervical cancer) is the most widely known.

Medium: cells are grown in chemically defined media which are balanced and buffered salt solutions with added amino acids and vitamins. Serum is always required—generally 10% (by volume) of calf serum (or sometimes fetal calf serum for delicate cells). Penicillin and streptomycin are included to prevent bacterial contamination.

Atmosphere: because the main buffer in the medium is bicarbonate, cells produce carbon dioxide: if this is lost to the air, e.g. in open petri plates, the pH of the medium becomes alkaline and kills the cells. Tissue cultures are therefore grown in stoppered test tubes or screw-capped bottles or, if in petri plates, in an incubator with the atmosphere enriched with 5 to 10% carbon dioxide.

Temperature: the optimal temperature is 37°C.

Specimens

Material from lesions or sites of infection usually collected on a wooden-shafted swab. The tip of the swab is broken off into a bottle of transport medium. Virus laboratories supply these on request.

Delivery: should be prompt as many viruses die off rapidly at room temperature. If delay is unavoidable, keep the specimen at 4°C (e.g. in a domestic refrigerator).

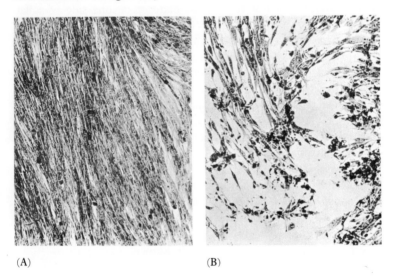

(A)   (B)

Fig. 3.5 CPE in a tissue culture of fibroblastic cells. (A) Uninoculated control. (B) Culture showing viral CPE.

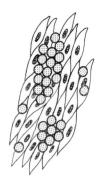

Fig. 3.6 Diagram of haemadsorption: clumps of erythrocytes are adhering to infected cells in the tissue culture.

Inoculation: a small volume of virus transport medium, fluid or an extract in buffer solution of the tissue or excretion, is added to the medium of a tube of tissue culture.

Virus growth is recognised by:

1. *CPE* (cytopathic effect): the virus kills the cells which round up and fall off the glass (Fig. 3.5). Some viruses cause cell fusion and their growth is recognised by the appearance of syncytia.
2. *Haemadsorption*: added erythrocytes adhere to the surface of infected cells with haemagglutinating virus (Fig. 3.6): sometimes virus can be detected by haemagglutination in the medium.
3. *Immunofluorescence*: infected cells are detected by fluorescence.

Identification: the virus isolated is identified serologically by neutralization of haemagglutination with standard antiviral serum: immunofluorescence (with standard or monoclonal antiviral antibody) or electron microscopy is also used.

2. Chick embryo

Rarely used now. Fig. 3.8 shows the main routes of inoculation.

Virus growth is recognised by the appearance of (i) pocks (or virus lesions) on the chorio-allantoic membrane or (ii) haemagglutinin in the amniotic or allantoic fluids (see Fig. 3.7).

3. Laboratory animals

Some viruses can only be isolated by inoculation of laboratory animals, usually mice. After inoculation the animals are observed

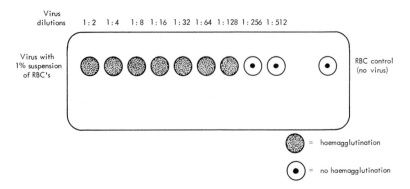

Fig. 3.7 Diagram of haemagglutination test for virus. Titre of virus haemagglutinin is 128.

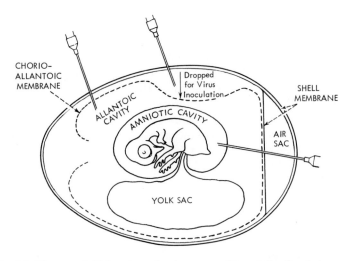

Fig. 3.8 Diagram of chick embryo showing routes of inoculation for viral isolation.

for signs of disease or death. The viruses are identified by testing for neutralization of their pathogenicity for animals by standard antiviral sera.

Direct demonstration of virus

This is now becoming a widely used—and fast—method of virus diagnosis. Virus or virus antigen is detected in lesions, fluids, tissues or excretions from the patient and a result can be obtained within an hour or two of receipt of the specimen. The main techniques are:

1. *Serological*: preferably with monoclonal antiviral antibody. The most popular method is immunofluorescence; ELIZA and radioimmune assay are now also being used for this.
2. *Electron microscopy*: virus particles are detected and can be provisionally identified (but not serologically typed) on the basis of their morphology.
3. *Probes*: Radioactive virus DNA can be used to detect virus genome or mRNA in tissues and fluids by molecular hybridization: still largely an experimental technique.

Inclusion bodies: are virus-induced masses seen in the nucleus or cytoplasm of infected cells. With a few exceptions they are too nonspecific to be useful in diagnosis.

4

Influenza

Influenza is one of the great epidemic diseases. From time to time, influenza becomes pandemic and sweeps throughout the world. The most severe pandemic recorded was in the winter of 1918 to 1919, when more than 20 million people perished. World-wide pandemics of influenza are due to the emergence of antigenically new strains of influenza virus to which there is no pre-existing immunity.

Clinical features

Route of infection: inhalation of respiratory secretions from an infected person.

Incubation period: from 1 to 4 days.

Signs and symptoms: fever, malaise, headache, generalized aches, sometimes with nasal discharge and sneezing; a non-productive hacking cough is common and there may be sore throat and hoarseness.

Duration: symptoms usually last for about 4 days but tiredness and weakness often persist for longer.

Primary site of virus multiplication: superficial epithelium of the upper and lower respiratory tract, influenza causes damage to the cilia and desquamation of the epithelium.

Complications

In a small proportion of cases, the acute infection progresses to pneumonia: two kinds of pneumonia may follow influenza:
1. *Primary influenzal pneumonia*, in which the condition of a patient

with typical influenza suddenly deteriorates with the onset of severe respiratory distress and symptoms of hypoxia, dyspnoea and cyanosis; circulatory collapse follows and the patient almost always dies. *Post mortem*, there is congestion of the lungs with desquamation of ciliated epithelium and hyperaemia of tracheal and bronchial mucosa; no significant bacteria are present.

2. *Secondary bacterial pneumonia*, usually developes later in the course of influenza and is due to secondary invasion of the lungs by bacteria such as *Staphylococcus aureus, Haemophilus influenzae* or pneumococci. The signs and symptoms are those of severe bacterial pneumonia; although there is a high mortality rate, the disease is less lethal than primary influenzal pneumonia. *Post mortem* there is heavy invasion of the lungs by bacteria.

Reye's syndrome

This is a rare complication mainly seen in children after influenza B (and other virus infections also); there is cerebral oedema and fatty degeneration of the viscera—especially the liver—which results in raised transaminase levels in the blood; there is a high mortality rate.

Types of virus

There are three influenza viruses, A, B and C, which can be differentiated by complement fixation test:

A—the principal cause of epidemic influenza;

B—usually associated with a milder disease but can also cause winter epidemics;

C—of doubtful pathogenicity for man.

Influenza A viruses are also found in animals—notably birds, pigs, and horses.

Epidemiology

Seasonal distribution: the highest incidence of infection is during the winter (but the epidemic of 'Asian' influenza started in Britain in the summer of 1957).

Spread: is more rapid than with any other infectious disease: in addition to other important properties, influenza virus possesses an inherent capacity for rapid spread.

Epidemics: pandemics of influenza A break out every few years and the epidemic strain spreads world-wide. The most severe epidemic with a high mortality rate was in 1918–19 and was due to a virus related to swine influenza A virus; unlike most influenza outbreaks this caused a high mortality amongst young adults: usually influenza is most severe in the elderly or in patients with chronic respiratory or cardiac disease.

Virology

1. Orthomyxoviruses ('myxo' = affinity for mucin).
2. RNA viruses—the RNA consists of eight separate fragments each of which codes for a different protein, e.g. the haemagglutinin, the neuraminidase, etc.
3. Roughly spherical particles, medium size, 80 to 100 nm, with an envelope which contains radially-projecting spikes of virus haemagglutinin and neuraminidase; inside the envelope is helically coiled nucleocapsid consisting of nucleoprotein i.e. RNA surrounded by protein capsomeres (Fig. 4.1).

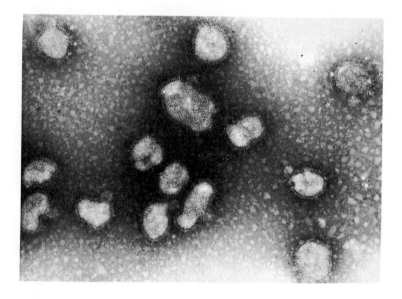

Fig. 4.1 Influenza virus. The virus nucleocapsid (or nucleic acid with protein capsid) has helical symmetry and is surrounded by an envelope containing spikes of haemagglutinin and neuraminidase × 90 000. (Photograph by Dr E.A.C. Follett.)

4. Haemagglutinate erythrocytes of various animal species.
5. Grow in amniotic cavity of the chick embryo and — after passage or subculture—in the allantoic cavity also.
6. Grow in monkey kidney tissue culture without CPE but with haemadsorption.

HAEMAGGLUTINATION BY INFLUENZA VIRUSES

Haemagglutination is due to adsorption of influenza virus particles to specific receptors on the erythrocyte surface.

Receptors are composed of muco-polysaccharide—neuraminic acid.

Virus haemagglutinin is contained in the envelope round the virus particle; the haemagglutinin has a combining site which is antigenic and has an affinity for neuraminic acid.

Neuraminidase. Influenza virus particles also contain an enzyme which is similar in action to the receptor destroying enzyme (RDE) of *Vibrio cholerae*; this destroys the neuraminic acid receptors on erythrocytes. After viral haemagglutination, if the mixture of virus and erythrocytes is kept at 37°C, the neuraminidase becomes active and causes the virus to elute from the erythrocytes; as a result the haemagglutination is reversed and the erythrocytes disperse again.

Haemagglutination-inhibition. Treatment of the virus with specific antibody prevents haemagglutination. Haemagglutination-inhibition is strain-specific, i.e. haemagglutination by a new virus strain, is unaffected by antibody to an influenza virus strain with a different haemagglutinin.

ANTIGENIC STRUCTURE

Influenza viruses have three main antigens:
1. '*S*' *or soluble antigen*—the protein in the ribonucleoprotein core of the virus particle: type specific in that all influenza A viruses share a common S antigen which is different to that shared by all influenza B viruses; demonstrated by complement fixation test.
2. *Haemagglutinin*: contained in the radially-projecting spikes in the virus envelope; strain-specific; the main neutralising antigen responsible for immunity to the virus.

3. *Neuraminidase*: also contained in the virus envelope; plays a minor role in immunity to reinfection.

Antigenic variation

Influenza viruses are unique among viruses in that they undergo antigenic change from time to time. Epidemics are due to the emergence of a new virus strain containing a haemagglutinin (and sometimes a neuraminidase also) different to those of previously circulating viruses so that the population has no herd immunity (i.e. antibody) to the new haemagglutinin.
Antigenic variation may be:
complete—*antigenic shift*
partial—*antigenic drift*

Antigenic shift: involves the replacement of the main neutralizing antigen—the haemagglutinin—by a different protein acquired as a result of genetic reassortment: the appropriate RNA segment which codes for the haemagglutinin is exchanged in one virus genome for another from a different, possibly animal, virus strain.

Antigenic shift is illustrated by the serological types of haemagglutinin and neuaminidase contained in the major influenza virus A strains which have circulated in the world during the past 40 years or so:

Year of emergence	Haemagglutinin	Neuraminidase
1918	H1	N1
1957	H2	N2
1968	H3	N2

Several pandemics of influenza have been recorded this century:
1. 1918–19: almost certainly due to a virus of which the haemagglutinin was similar to one commonly found in swine influenza strains
2. 1934: the first influenza virus was isolated
3. 1957: H2N2—the 'Asian flu' epidemic
4. 1968: H3N2—the 'Hong Kong flu' epidemic
5. 1977: H1N1 reappeared—'Red flu'—but caused infection only in young people under 20 years of age—because older people had antibody from exposure to the virus before 1957.

At present: both H3N2 and H1N1 strains have circulated together in countries throughout the world since 1977.

Antigenic drift is due to minor changes in the amino acid sequence of the haemagglutinin protein (but the haemagglutinin remains basically the same protein). The changes are the result of spontaneous mutations; the mutant strain of virus becomes selected in the population by its ability to infect partially immune hosts: antigenic drift increases progressively from season to season.

Influenza B
Also shows antigenic variation but the changes are less dramatic than with influenza A.
1. 1973: a new strain B/Hong Kong/5/73 appeared.
2. 1979: B/Singapore/222/79 appeared.

At present: circulating strains show considerable heterogeneity but generally resemble the 1979 virus more closely than the 1973 strain.

Diagnosis

Serology (the most widely used)

Complement fixation test: with the 'S' or soluble antigen

Isolation

Specimen: mouth washings and throat swabs

Inoculate
1. Monkey kidney tissue cultures
   (i) *Observe* for haemagglutination or haemadsorption of human group O erythrocytes.
   (ii) *Virus is typed* by haemagglutination-inhibition with specific antisera.
2. Amniotic cavity of chick embryo (now rarely used)
   (i) *Observe* for haemagglutination of fowl erythrocytes.
   (ii) *Virus is typed* by testing for inhibition of haemagglutination with standard antisera.

Direct demonstration
Specimen: naso-pharyngeal aspirate.

Detect virus antigen by indirect immunofluorescence.

Vaccines

At the time of a pandemic, the speed with which new strains of influenza virus spread makes it difficult if not impossible to prepared sufficient quantities of vaccine in time to protect any but a few key workers.

Inactivated virus vaccines

Administered by subcutaneous injection; saline suspension of purified virus or virus subunits (i.e. haemagglutinin and neuraminidase) grown in the allantoic cavity of the chick embryo.

In general, influenza vaccines give relatively short-lived immunity—usually lasting only a few months. At best the protection conferred is of the order of 60%.

Guillain-Barré syndrome: a polyneuritis with ascending paralysis usually starting in the legs is a rare complication of influenza vaccine: clears up spontaneously although positive pressure respiration may be required during the acute phase due to paralysis of the respiratory muscles.

Live attenuated virus vaccines

Administered intra-nasally: not yet generally accepted.

5

Upper respiratory tract infections

The classification of respiratory tract infections as 'upper' or 'lower' is an over-simplification as most respiratory viruses can infect both upper and lower respiratory tracts. Predominately upper respiratory syndromes often show some involvement of the lower respiratory tract and vice versa.

Respiratory infections are a major problem in medicine because of their frequency, and are of considerable economic importance because they cause so much absence from work. So far, there is no foreseeable prospect of controlling these infections; most spread rapidly by inhalation of infected respiratory secretions.

The principal viruses which primarily affect the upper respiratory tract are shown in Table 5.1.

Table 5.1 Viruses which affect the upper respiratory tract

Virus	No. of serotypes	Disease
Parainfluenza viruses	4	croup; colds, lower respiratory infections in children
Respiratory syncytial virus	1	bronchiolitis and pneumonia in infants, colds in older children
Rhinoviruses	100+	colds
Adenoviruses	41	pharyngitis and conjunctivitis
Coronaviruses	3	colds
Coxsackieviruses	types A21, B3	colds
Echoviruses	types 11, 20	colds

PARAINFLUENZA VIRUSES

Clinical features

Febrile common cold: with sore throat, hoarseness and cough.

Croup or acute laryngo-tracheobronchitis: characterized by hoarseness and cough; in infants, the disease may be very severe with respiratory distress, inspiratory stridor and cyanosis requiring tracheostomy.

Bronchiolitis and pneumonia in young children are also sometimes caused by parainfluenza viruses.

Age. Both children and adults but infection is most common in children under 5 years old; the more severe lower respiratory tract infections are seen mainly in pre-school children.

Serotypes. There are 4 parainfluenza viruses—types 1, 2, 3 and 4— but type 4 is of lower pathogenicity.

Serotypes and disease. Although there is considerable overlap, type 3 virus is particularly associated with bronchiolitis and bronchopneumonia and types 1 and 2 with croup. Type 3 infects younger children than types 1 and 2.

Epidemiology. Parainfluenza viruses cause disease all year round but type 3 causes outbreaks of infection every year in the summer and autumn; type 1 outbreaks in contrast are less frequent—usually every 2 years.

Virology

1. Paramyxoviruses
2. RNA viruses
3. Large enveloped particles, 100 to 200 nm, with helical symmetry possessing both a haemagglutinin and a neuraminidase
4. Haemagglutinate human group O erythrocytes
5. Grow in monkey kidney tissue cultures with haemadsorption.

Diagnosis

Isolation

Specimens: mouth washings, throat swabs.

Inoculate: monkey kidney tissue cultures.

Observe: for haemadsorption with human group O erythrocytes (CPE is variable and slow) or immunofluorescence.

Type virus: by neutralisation test of haemadsorption by standard antisera.

Serology
Of limited value.

RESPIRATORY SYNCYTIAL VIRUS

Respiratory syncytial virus causes common colds but its importance lies in its tendency to invade the lower respiratory tract in infants under 1 year old causing bronchiolitis or pneumonia.

Clinical features

Bronchiolitis usually starts with nasal obstruction and discharge followed by fever, cough, rapid breathing, expiratory wheezes and signs of respiratory distress such as cyanosis and inspiratory indrawing of the intercostal spaces.

Pneumonia: in respiratory syncytial virus pneumonia there is a similar clinical picture with fever, cyanosis, prostration and rapid breathing but without expiratory wheezing.

Bronchiolitis and pneumonia are severe diseases with a mortality rate of from 2 to 5 per cent.

Immunopathology. Inactivated vaccine against this virus enhanced the incidence of bronchiolitis and pneumonia in vaccinees compared to controls; since the diseases appear mainly in infants in whom maternal antibody is still present, it seemed probable that both diseases might be partly *immunological*, e.g. due to the formation of immune complexes. Alternatively, the susceptibility of very young infants of these diseases may be *mechanical* and caused by the narrowness of the bronchiolar lumen: when this is inflamed, serious obstruction may be produced more readily than in older infants with wider bronchioles. This second explanation is now the more widely accepted.

Common colds. Respiratory syncytial virus also causes common colds without lower respiratory tract involvement: these are seen in older children and—rarely—in adults as well as infants.

Age. Bronchiolitis and pneumonia are almost confined to infants under one year old and are most common in those aged less than 6 months; common colds due to respiratory syncytial virus are mainly seen in pre-school children.

Epidemiology

Every year there are outbreaks of respiratory syncytial virus during the later winter months especially from February to April.

Virology

1. Pneumovirus—within the paramyxovirus family, one serological type
2. RNA virus
3. Pleomorphic enveloped particles, medium size, 90 to 130 nm; helical symmetry (Fig. 5.1)

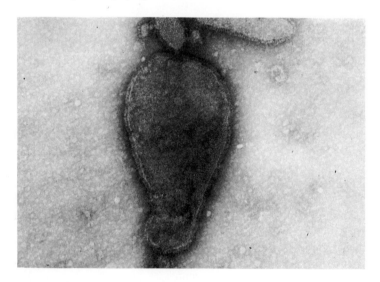

Fig. 5.1 Respiratory syncytial virus. Pleomorphic virus with helical nucleocapsid surrounded by an envelope. × 90 000. (Photograph by Dr E A C Follett.)

4. Grows in cells with syncytial CPE
5. Does not haemagglutinate.

Diagnosis

Direct demonstration of virus in nasopharyngeal aspirates by immunofluorescence.

Isolation

Specimens: mouth washings, nasal secretions (not frozen during delivery because the virus is inactivated by freezing).

Inoculate: HeLa cells (Bristol strain), HEp-2 cells.

Observe: for characteristic CPE of syncytia of multinucleated giant cells.

Type virus: by immunofluorescence or by complement fixation test with standard antiserum.

Serology
Complement fixation test

RHINOVIRUSES

Rhinoviruses are the main cause of common colds—the most common of all infectious diseases and by far the most frequent form of respiratory infection.

Clinical features

Incubation period: 2 to 4 days.

Signs and symptoms. Nasal discharge with nasal obstruction, sneezing, sore throat and cough; about half the patients are mildly febrile; hoarseness and headache are common especially in adults.

Duration. On average symptoms subside in about a week but are prolonged for up to 2 weeks in a proportion of cases; complications are rare.

Spread. Rhinoviruses may also spread by contact (i.e. from hand to nose) as well as by inhalation of respiratory secretions.

Age. Infections are most frequent in pre-school children; thereafter the attack rate falls but infections remain common even amongst adults.

Incidence. The reported attack rate for rhinovirus infections varies in different reports but on average the attack rate is about 0.7 rhinovirus infections per person per year.

Seasonal incidence. Infections are found all year round but the incidence is highest in autumn and winter.

Immunity. Neutralising antibody is formed after rhinovirus infection and this has a protective effect against re-infection with the particular serotype responsible.

Epidemiology

This is complex as would be expected from the large number of different virus serotypes. In any community at a given time, several serotypes can be found circulating; over a long period of time, however, there is a gradual change in the serotypes present possibly due to increasing immunity within the population to earlier serotypes.

Virology

1. Picornaviruses (pico = small + RNA); more than 100 serotypes (there is some evidence that rhinoviruses may undergo antigenic variation).
2. RNA viruses
3. Small, icosahedral particles, 22 to 30 nm
4. Inactivated at acid pH (unlike enteroviruses—the other members of the picornavirus group)
5. Grow in tissue cultures but at 33°C, instead of the usual 37°C (the temperature of the nostrils is 33°C)
6. Two groups of viruses:
   a. 'M' rhinoviruses grow in monkey kidney tissue culture with CPE

b. 'H' rhinoviruses grow only in human embryo cells—with CPE: a larger group than the 'M' viruses.

Diagnosis

Isolation

Specimens: nasal secretions, mouth washings.

Inoculate: human embryo lung and monkey kidney cell cultures.

Observe: for CPE.

Type virus: by neutralisation with standard antisera.

Serology
Impractical because of the large number of serological types of rhinovirus.

Note: Laboratory diagnosis of common colds is too time-consuming for routine purposes and is therefore restricted to epidemiological research.

ADENOVIRUSES

Clinical features

Clinically, the main symptoms of adenovirus respiratory infection are *pharyngitis and conjunctivitis*. The main syndromes are usually classified as shown in Table 5.2.

Table 5.2 Syndromes associated with adenoviruses

Syndrome	Adenovirus types
1. *Epidemic infection* pharyngo-conjunctival fever, acute respiratory disease	3, 4, 7, 14, 21
2. *Endemic infection* pharyngitis, follicular conjunctivitis	1 2, 3, 5, 6, 7
3. *Epidemic kerato-conjunctivitis or 'shipyard eye'*	8

1. *Epidemic infection*: common in recruit camps where attack rates of 70 per cent have been reported; also seen in children's institutions due to crowding together of susceptible young hosts.

2. *Endemic infection*: adenovirus infections are endemic but at a low level in the general population: they usually constitute less than 5 per cent of the respiratory infections in the community at large; types 1, 2, 5 and 6 are associated with endemic infection, but cases of infection due to types 3 and 7 are common in the community and tend to be found in clusters.

3. *Epidemic kerato-conjunctivitis*: a form of eye infection which is spread mainly by contaminated instruments at eye clinics and surgeries; epidemics are seen in eye patients and also in shipyard and metal workers who are prone to minor eye injuries which require treatment at eye clinics: unlike the other forms of adeno-virus disease, this disease is mainly associated with adenovirus type 8.

Alimentary tract: adenoviruses are common in the alimentary as well as the respiratory tract; this is probably due to their predilection for lymphoid tissue; adenoviruses may play a role in mesenteric adenitis and possibly intussusception in children.

Oncogenic properties: several adenoviruses cause cancer on injection into hamsters; the most highly oncogenic are types 12, 18 and 31. However, adenoviruses do not cause tumours in man.

Chronic infection: adenoviruses have a tendency to persist for long periods in tissues such as the tonsils and adenoids: this may not be true latency but rather a low grade persistent infection.

Virology

1. 41 serological types which react independently in neutralisation tests but share a common group complement fixing antigen.
2. DNA viruses.
3. Medium size: 60 to 70 nm; icosahedron-shaped particles with cubic symmetry and with fibres topped with knobs projecting from the vertices (Fig. 5.2).
4. Most haemagglutinate.
5. Grow slowly in tissue cultures, (human embryonic cells or HeLa cells are best) with CPE of clusters of rounded and 'ballooned' cells.

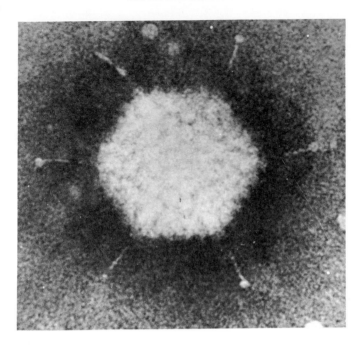

Fig. 5.2 Adenovirus. Icosahedron particle with cubic symmetry and fibres which project from the vertices. × 200 000. (Reproduced, with permission, from Valentine, R C & Pereira, H G, 1965, *Journal of Molecular Biology*, **13**, 13

Diagnosis

Isolation

Specimens: mouth washings, throat swabs, faeces.

Inoculate: human embryonic cell cultures or HeLa cells.

Observe: for characteristic CPE of large rounded cells arranged like 'bunches of grapes'.

Type virus by neutralisation test.

Serology
Complement fixation test detects antibody to adenovirus group antigen but not the serotype of the advenovirus responsible.

OTHER VIRUSES CAUSING COMMON COLDS

Coronaviruses

Medium sized (80 to 100 nm) RNA viruses; characteristic enveloped particles surrounded by a fringe of club-shaped projections; haemagglutinate: can only be isolated in organ cultures of human embryo trachea although some strains have been adapted to growth in the L 132 line of human embryo lung cells with CPE. There are at least 3 antigenic types although with some antigenic cross-reactions or sharing between the types.

Coronaviruses cause from 2 to 10% of colds in the community but the difficulty of isolating them in the laboratory means that they are seldom diagnosed.

Enteroviruses

Some enteroviruses cause respiratory infections; the main types associated with respiratory disease are Coxsackievirus A21 (Coe virus), B3 and echovirus types 11 and 20).

6

Neurological disease due to viruses

Neurological disease is a serious and not uncommon complication of virus infection. Most human pathogenic viruses are capable of spreading to the central nervous system (CNS).

Virus lesions in the CNS are due mainly to *viral multiplication* in the cells of the nervous tissues with cellular damage and dysfunction and consequent neurological signs and symptoms. But the *immune response of the host* may also play a role in causing lesions. In one form of viral CNS disease (post-infectious encephalomyelitis) virus cannot be isolated from the CNS.

Spread: most viruses invade the CNS *by the blood stream* but some, e.g. rabies, reach the CNS by the *neural route* by spreading along the peripheral nerves.

CNS involvement is not always followed by neurological disease—for example there is evidence that *symptomless involvement of the CNS* is common in measles and mumps.

Virus neurological diseases fall into two clinical categories—acute and chronic.

ACUTE VIRAL NEUROLOGICAL DISEASE:

There are four main syndromes:
1. *Encephalitis*. The main symptoms are drowsiness, mental confusion, convulsions, focal neurological signs and sometimes coma
2. *Paralysis*. With fever, flaccid paralysis—most often of the lower limbs—and signs of meningitis such as headache with stiffness of neck and back
3. *Aseptic meningitis*. A relatively mild disease with fever, headache and stiffness of neck and back

Table 6.1 Acute virus neurological diseases

	Direct invasion of CNS by virus		Virus not demonstrable in CNS (disease is probably due to abnormal immune response of host to infection)
Disease	Encephalitis	Paralysis (poliomyelitis)	Aseptic meningitis	Post-infectious encephalomyelitis
Site	Brain	Anterior horn cells of spinal cord	Meninges	Brain
Lesions	Destructive lesions in grey matter; neuronal damage	Destructive lesions of lower motor neurones with meningitis	Inflammation of meninges, cells in CSF (usually lymphocytes)	Perivascular infiltration, microglial proliferation, demyelination
Viruses	Herpes simplex, arboviruses rabies	Enteroviruses (especially polioviruses)	Enteroviruses, mumps, lymphocytic chorio-meningitis	Measles, rubella, varicella-zoster vaccinia

Table 6.2 Chronic virus neurological diseases

Disease	Subacute sclerosing panencephalitis	Progressive multifocal leucoencephalopathy	Kuru	Creutzfeldt Jakob disease
Site	Brain	Brain	Brain	Brain and spinal cord
Lesions	Neuronal degeneration, intranuclear inclusions	Multiple foci of degeneration	Spongiform degeneration especially in cerebellum	Spongiform degeneration
Viruses	Measles, rubella (after congenital infection)	JC virus	Transmissible by filter-passing agent	Transmissible by filter-passing agent

4. *Post-infectious encephalomyelitis* (also called encephalitis). Symptoms are similar to those of encephalitis.

Table 6.1 summarises the principal features of the four main acute viral neurological syndromes.

CHRONIC VIRUS NEUROLOGICAL DISEASES

Viruses cause several chronic neurological diseases which are listed in Table 6.2. The diseases are described in more detail in the chapters on the viruses which cause them but below are some of the main features:

1. *Rare*. All the disease are very rare and most doctors will never see a case of any of them throughout their working lives
2. *Signs and symptoms*. Numerous and varied but are neurological and often affect intellectual capacity as well as both motor and sensory functions
3. *Duration*. The diseases may last for months or even years but are relentlessly progressive
4. *Fatal*. The diseases are always fatal.

7

Enterovirus infections; infantile gastroenteritis

Enteroviruses are a large family of viruses, of which the main site of infection is the gut; nevertheless, they rarely cause intestinal symptoms; enterovirus diseases are the result of spread of the viruses to other sites in the body—particularly the CNS.

Below are listed the various groups included in the enterovirus family:

		Enteroviruses			
		*Coxsackieviruses**		*echoviruses***	*enteroviruses (unclassified)*
		group A	*group B*		
types	1–3	1–24	1–6	1–34	68–72***

    * Coxsackie is the village in New York where these viruses were first isolated.
    ** Enteric, Cytopathic, Human, Orphan (because originally—but wrongly—thought not to be associated with human disease).
    *** Enterovirus 72 is hepatitis A virus (see Chapter 13)

Enteroviruses have the following properties:
Enter the body via ingestion by mouth.
Primary site of multiplication is the lymphoid tissue of the alimentary tract—including the pharynx.
Spread from the gut is in two directions:
1. *Outwards* into the blood (viraemia) and so to other tissues and organs
2. *Inwards* into the lumen of the gut and to excretion in the faeces.

Clinical features

The main enterovirus diseases are shown in Table 7.1.

Table 7.1 Enterovirus disease

Syndrome	Main viruses responsible
1. Neurological	
(i) Paralysis	polioviruses
(ii) Aseptic meningitis	most enteroviruses
2. Febrile illness	most enteroviruses
3. Herpangina; hand, foot and mouth disease	Coxsackie A viruses
4. Myocarditis, pericarditis	Coxsackie B viruses
5. Bornholm disease	Coxsackie B viruses
6. Acute haemorrhagic conjunctivitis	enterovirus 70

General features of enterovirus infections: most enterovirus infections are confined to the alimentary tract and are symptomless: enteroviruses do not cause diarrhoea

A small proportion of infections give rise to febrile illness due to viraemia.

A few cases progress to aseptic meningitis but spread of virus to the CNS or other organs and tissues is a rare complication of enterovirus infection.

NEUROLOGICAL SYNDROMES

Neurological disease is the most important manifestation of enteroviral infection; it is not associated with one particular group or type of enterovirus.

The illness is usually biphasic: the initial symptoms are of a febrile illness due to viraemia; there is an intervening period of well-being for a day or two followed by the onset of neurological symptoms; these are due to spread of the virus through the 'blood-brain barrier' to invade the CNS.

There are two main types of neurological disease due to enteroviruses:

1. *Paralysis* or poliomyelitis: an acute illness with pain and *flaccid* paralysis affecting mainly the lower legs. Sometimes the muscles of respiration become involved requiring tracheostomy with

controlled breathing by positive-pressure respirator: more rarely, the disease may take the form of *bulbar paralysis* when the muscles of breathing and swallowing are primarily involved. Paralysis is an extension of aseptic meningitis and is therefore accompanied by the signs and symptoms of that syndrome.

Pathology: paralysis is due to viral damage to the cells of the anterior horn of the spinal cord with lower motor neurone lesions resulting in flaccid paralysis. If damage to the nerve cells is severe, the paralysis may be permanent.

Paralysis is most often due to the three polioviruses and especially poliovirus 1. Before the introduction of poliovaccine, epidemics of paralysis were common in countries with a high standard of living e.g. USA, Denmark and Australia.

2. *Aseptic meningitis*: signs of neurological disease are present but the damage is minor and there is no paralysis; the main signs and symptoms are fever and headache with nuchal rigidity (stiffness of the neck muscles due to meningeal irritation). Lymphocytes and protein in the cerebrospinal fluid (CSF) are increased. The prognosis is good and most patients recover completely.

Epidemics of aseptic meningitis are common: often due to echovirus 9 or, before widespread use of poliovaccine, to polioviruses; echoviruses 4, 6, 11, 14, 16 and 30 and Coxsackieviruses A7, A9 and B5 have also caused epidemic aseptic meningitis.

NON-NEUROLOGICAL SYNDROMES

Febrile illness: a common manifestation of enterovirus infection with viraemia.

Rash: many enteroviruses cause rash but this is particularly common with Coxsackie A9 and A16 (see below) and echovirus 9.

Herpangina: a painful eruption of vesicles in the mouth and throat: recently, it has been reported as part of the syndrome of 'hand, foot and mouth disease' in which there are vesicles also on the hands and feet; due to group A Coxsackieviruses (especially A16); enterovirus 71 has also caused hand, foot and mouth disease.

Bornholm disease: also known as pleurodynia or epidemic myalgia: a painful inflammation of muscles which mainly involves the intercostal muscles. The disease is named after the Danish island where there was an extensive outbreak in 1930; due to group B Coxsackieviruses.

Myocarditis and pericarditis: due to Group B Coxsackieviruses. *Myocarditis* is characterized by rapid pulse, enlargement of the heart and ECG abnormalities and *pericarditis* by pericardial friction or effusion.

Each syndrome can be present on its own but patients often develop myocarditis and pericarditis together. Both diseases are seen mainly in adult males, and may be mistaken for myocardial infarction; however, the prognosis is good and most patients recover completely. Rarely epidemics have been reported among neonates in hospital nurseries. In the 1965 epidemic of Coxsackievirus B5 infections in England and Wales, 15% of the patients had cardiac signs or symptoms the incidence being higher in adults than in children.

Acute haemorrhagic conjunctivitis: due to enterovirus 70 has appeared in large-scale outbreaks in 1969–71 in Africa, South-East Asia, Japan, India and, to a limited extent, in Britain. The incubation period is 24 hours and the disease lasts about 10 days: patients recover completely: the disease spreads rapidly, probably via eye discharges. Unlike most enterovirus infections the causal virus is not found in the faeces.

Epidemiology

Enterovirus infections are common—especially in children and in conditions of poor hygiene.

Infection is spread mainly by the faecal-oral route from virus excretors to contacts; virus in pharyngeal secretions may also be a source of infection.

Gut immunity: after infection with an enterovirus, the gut becomes resistant to reinfection with the same virus; this resistance is due to the production in the gut of virus-specific neutralising IgA antibody.

Seasonal distribution: infections are more frequent in the summer than in the winter months.

Predominant strains: one or two enterovirus types usually predominate in a season; the types which emerge are determined by the level of immunity in the population concerned; this in turn depends on the previous infections experienced by the community.

Poor sanitation, e.g. in under-developed countries, increases the chances of childhood infection so that immunity is acquired early in life.

High standard of living in countries such as the USA, diminishes the chance of infection and therefore of immunity being acquired in childhood.

Adults are more liable to develop severe paralysis in poliovirus infection than children: the risk of this is increased by pregnancy, tonsillectomy, fatigue, trauma or inoculation with bacterial vaccines.

Epidemics: countries with a high standard of living have a relatively large proportion of non-immune adults and before the advent of poliovaccines suffered from repeated and widespread epidemics of paralytic disease.

Virology

1. Picornaviruses (pico = small + RNA):
2. RNA viruses
3. Small roughly spherical particles, 25 to 30 nm (Fig. 7.1)
4. Stable at acid pH (in contrast to the rhinoviruses—the other members of the picornavirus group)
5. Most grow in tissue cultures with rapid production of CPE
6. Coxsackieviruses (but not polio or echoviruses) are pathogenic for suckling mice.

Diagnosis

Isolation

Specimens: faeces, throat swabs: CSF is useful for some viruses (e.g. echovirus 9) but not for polioviruses.

Inoculate: monkey kidney, human embryo lung or RD cell cultures.

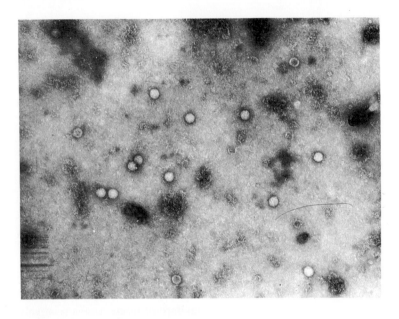

Fig. 7.1 Echovirus. All enteroviruses look like this with very small virus particles with cubic symmetry. × 90 000. (Photograph by Dr E. A. C. Follett.)

Observe: for CPE.

Type virus: by neutralisation tests with standard antisera; usually done using pooled antisera to reduce the number of tests.

Note: Most Coxsackie A viruses do not grow in tissue cultures so if Coxsackie A virus infection is suspected:

Inoculate: suckling mice subcutaneously and intracerebrally.

Observe: for characteristic signs of disease.
   Group A coxsackieviruses cause flaccid paralysis due to widespread myositis.
Note: Group B Coxsackieviruses cause spastic paralysis with tremor due to cerebral lesions and fat-pad necrosis.

Serology
Neutralisation tests are useful for the diagnosis of poliomyelitis and Coxsackie B virus infections.

Apart from this, the large number of enteroviruses make serological diagnosis impracticable.

Vaccination

Two vaccines are available against the most paralytogenic enteroviruses, i.e. the three polioviruses.

1. Sabin live attenuated virus vaccine
Now the main vaccine used for poliomyelitis immunisation.

Contains the three polioviruses as attenuated strains which have lost neurovirulence for monkeys (i.e. ability to produce paralysis or lesions in CNS of monkeys); grown in monkey kidney tissue cultures.

Administered in three oral doses along with triple vaccine starting at 6 months of age: booster at age 15 to 19 years when leaving school

Protection: good.

Blood antibody response: good.

Gut immunity: good, vaccinated children show increased resistance to alimentary infection; this is due to the appearance of virus-specific IgA in the gut produced in response to the vaccine.

Safety: good; very rarely paralysis—usually mild and usually due to the type 3 component: incidence about 1 per million doses.

Vaccinated children are infectious to others so that vaccine strains may circulate to some extent in the community.

Widespread use of this vaccine has resulted in a dramatic decrease both in paralytic poliomyelitis and in the circulation of wild polioviruses in the community.

2. Salk inactivated virus vaccine
This was the first polio vaccine to be used on a large scale but has now been largely replaced by Sabin vaccine. It contains the three polioviruses inactivated by formaldehyde and is given in three

injections. Although producing good blood antibody levels—and therefore good protection against paralysis—it fails to give gut immunity.

INFANTILE GASTROENTERITIS

Also known as acute non-bacterial gastroenteritis, this disease causes acute diarrhoea in infants; in Britain today the disease is generally mild but is an important cause of infant mortality in under-developed countries. Several viruses are implicated but the main cause of the disease is rotavirus. Rotavirus is a genus within the reovirus family (i.e. viruses with a fragmented double-stranded RNA genome and a double layered capsid).

Clinical features

Incubation period: 1 to 4 days.

Symptoms: Acute onset of vomiting—which is sometimes projectile—and diarrhoea; dehydration is common and may require intravenous fluid replacement as a life-saving emergency procedure: respiratory symptoms e.g. cough, coryza, are common.

Duration: About a week.

Age: Most common in infants—especially in babies less than one year old; although rarer, cases have been reported in adults.

Epidemics are common especially amongst babies in nurseries.

Seasonal: infections are more common in winter than summer.

Virus is excreted in faeces during the acute stage of illness.

Virology

1. Reovirus family
2. RNA—double-stranded, in 11 fragments.
3. Particles with cubic symmetry, 65 nm diameter with a characteristic wheel-like appearance of their two-layered capsid (Fig. 7.2).
4. Two (probably more) serological types
5. Does not grow in tissue culture.

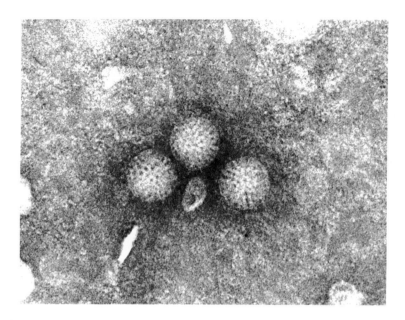

Fig. 7.2 Rotavirus. Spherical particles with cubic symmetry, showing characteristic outer layer like the spokes of a wheel which distinguishes the virus from reovirus. × 200 000. (Photograph by Prof. C. R. Madeley.)

Diagnosis

Demonstration of virus by:
1. Electron microscopy to detect typical virus particles in faecal samples.
2. Serological tests for virus antigen in faeces by complement fixation or ELISA tests.

Other viruses causing gastroenteritis

Many morphologically distinct viruses have been detected in the stools of children with diarrhoea:
1. Caliciviruses
2. Astroviruses
3. Adenoviruses (most do not grow in tissue culture unlike their respiratory counterparts)
4. Small round viruses
5. Norwalk agent

Their significance as a cause of gastroenteritis is uncertain: Norwalk agent and related viruses have been found in outbreaks in the USA.

Winter vomiting disease: a syndrome of acute vomiting but variable diarrhoea (the symptoms overlap with those of acute gastroenteritis): caliciviruses may be responsible for some outbreaks.

8

Arthropod-borne virus infections

Many virus diseases are transmitted by the bite of an arthropod vector. The viruses are called *arboviruses* and multiply in the bodies of arthropods.

Arboviruses are extremely numerous and include many unrelated viruses belonging to different virus groups:

1. *Togaviruses*
   Subdivided into:
   a. *Alphaviruses* (formerly group A arboviruses)
   b. *Flaviviruses*
2. *Bunyaviruses*
   Subdivided into
   a. *Bunyaviruses*
   b. *Phleboviruses*
3. *Orbiviruses*
   A subdivision of the reovirus family.

Vectors: Mosquitoes, ticks and sandflies are the principal arthropod vectors which transmit arboviruses.

Animal hosts. The main reservoirs are wild birds and small mammals; the viruses spread to man when an arthropod vector acquires virus from its natural host and transmits it in the course of biting the human host.

Disease. Arboviruses cause two main types of disease:
1. Encephalitis
2. Fever (often with haemorrhage)

Some of the most important arboviruses are listed in Table 8.1 together with their vectors and the diseases they produce.

ARBOVIRUS ENCEPHALITIS

Arbovirus encephalitis is a world-wide problem. It is common in North and South America (Eastern, Western and Venezuelan equine encephalitis, Rociovirus, California and St Louis encephalitis), the Far East (Japanese B encephalitis), Eastern Europe (tick-borne encephalitis) and Australia (Murray Valley encephalitis). It is not a problem in Britain where the only arbovirus found is th͏ causing the tick-borne disease, louping ill, in sheep—and on͏ occasionally in man.

Table 8.1 Classification of arboviruses

Virus	Disease	Vector
Alphaviruses		
Eastern equine encephalitis	Encephalitis	Mosquito
Western equine encephalitis	Encephalitis	Mosquito
Venezuelan equine	Encephalitis,	
encephalitis	febrile disease	Mosquito
Chikungunya	Febrile disease	Mosquito
Ross River	Febrile disease	Mosquito
Flaviviruses		
St Louis encephalitis	Encephalitis	Mosquito
Japanese B encephalitis	Encephalitis	Mosquito
Murray Valley encephalitis	Encephalitis	Mosquito
Tick-borne encephalitis	Encephalitis	Tick
Yellow fever	Haemorrhagic fever	Mosquito
Rocio	Encephalitis	Mosquito
Kyasanur Forest Fever	Haemorrhagic fever	Tick
Dengue	Febrile disease haemorrhagic fever	Mosquito
Bunyaviruses		
California encephalitis	Encephalitis	Mosquito
Congo/Crimean haemorrhagic fever	Haemorrhagic fever	Tick
Oropouche	Febrile disease	Midge
Phlebovirus		
Rift Valley fever	Febrile disease haemorrhagic fever	Mosquito
Orbivirus		
Colorado tick fever	Febrile disease	Tick

Clinically, the main symptoms are fever, progressively severe headache, nausea, vomiting, stiffness of neck, back and legs; there may be convulsions, drowsiness, deepening coma or neurological signs such as paralysis and tremor.

Symptomless infection is common with most of the arboviruses which cause encephalitis. After an epidemic, arbovirus antibodies are present in a considerable proportion of the population; the incidence of encephalitis as a result of arbovirus infection is usually low although some viruses, e.g. Eastern equine encephalitis virus, cause symptoms in a higher proportion of people infected than others, e.g. Venezuelan equine encephalitis. Eastern equine encephalitis also has a higher mortality rate.

Age. Arbovirus encephalitis affects all ages although some variations are seen with different viruses. For example, California encephalitis is mainly seen in school children whereas St Louis encephalitis produces its most severe effects in older people in whom neurological sequelae are common; Western equine encephalitis on the other hand produces more sequelae in young people.

Epidemics of arbovirus encephalitis are common and have been well studied in the USA: epidemics are seasonal, infection being more frequent in summer and autumn. Before and during a human epidemic there is evidence of infection spreading in the animals, e.g. birds, that are the natural hosts of the virus; in Eastern, Western and Venezuelan equine encephalitis, epidemics of human infection are preceded by, or concurrent, with epidemic infection in horses. The horses, like man, are secondary hosts of the viruses, the primary or natural hosts being birds (Eastern and Western) and small mammals (Venezuelan).

ARBOVIRUS FEVERS AND HAEMORRHAGIC FEVERS

These syndromes overlap to some extent in that haemorrhages are not infrequent complications of arbovirus fevers; there is some evidence that the haemorrhagic forms of disease may be due to formation of immune complexes due to abnormally large production of antibodies.

Note: haemorrhagic fevers are also caused by other, non-arthropod-borne viruses (see Chapter 9).

Epidemiology. Worldwide in distribution especially in semi-tropical and tropical countries; epidemics are frequent and are a major health problem. Symptomless infection—detected by a relatively high incidence of antibodies in the general population concerned—is common.

Clinically, the symptoms are those of a severe generalized febrile disease with high fever, chills, severe headache, pain in the limbs, nausea and vomiting; some arbovirus fevers have additional signs and symptoms such as rash or arthritis.

Below are some of the best known arbovirus fevers:

Yellow fever
Endemic in South America and the central belt of Africa. There are two forms:
1. *Urban* in which the reservoir of the virus is man and the vector the mosquito *Aedes aegypti*.
2. *Sylvan or jungle* in which the reservoir is tree-dwelling monkeys and the vector various species of forest mosquito.

Clinically, the most striking feature of yellow fever is jaundice due to viral invasion of the liver causing hepatitis; haemorrhages are often seen and a toxic nephrosis with proteinuria is a common feature.

Kyasanur Forest fever
A haemorrhagic fever seen mainly in forest workers in Mysore State, India: the animal reservoirs are monkeys and possibly small mammals also.

Dengue
Dengue is a major health problem in South-east Asia, India, the Pacific Islands, and the Caribbean; infection is widespread in these areas; monkeys are probably the main reservoir of infection and the main vector is *Aedes aegypti*.

Antigenic types: there are four sub-types (types 1 to 4) of dengue virus.

Clinically, dengue typically presents the classical features of a severe febrile disease with pain in the limbs and rash; the case fatality rate of this type of dengue is low.

Dengue haemorrhagic shock syndrome: a serious complication of dengue in young children. In this syndrome, an attack of dengue progresses to a more severe disease characterized by haemorrhages and shock; seen in children who have experienced a previous attack of dengue due to a different sub-type of virus: on re-infection with the second virus, immune complexes are formed due to production of excess antibody; the immune complexes with complement activation are responsible for the haemorrhagic shock syndrome.

Chikunguna (and the similar and related virus O'nyong-nyong)

The cause of widespread epidemics of febrile disease in Africa and Asia.

Clinically, both diseases are characterized by severe pain in the joints: O'nyong-nyong is a dialect name meaning break-bone fever. Residual joint pains may persist after recovery from the acute disease.

Haemorrhagic fever: both diseases sometimes cause haemorrhagic fever and, occasionally, shock syndrome.

Ross River virus

The cause of epidemics in Australia and the Pacific of febrile disease with rash and polyarthritis.

Congo/Crimean haemorrhagic fever

This is seen in Southern Russia, Bulgaria and in West and East Africa: more recently the disease has been reported in the Middle East and Pakistan: can also apread case-to-case to medical and nursing staff via contact with infected blood.

Clinically, the disease has a high mortality rate: the most serious cases show a marked haemorrhagic tendency sometimes with extensive skin ecchymoses. There is evidence that severely haemorrhagic cases have a greater antibody response than patients with milder disease.

Oropouche

This bunyavirus has caused epidemics of mild febrile disease, sometimes with rash and sometimes with meningitis, in Brazil.

Rift Valley fever

Responsible for large epizootics in sheep and cattle in Africa—particularly Egypt, the Sudan and South Africa. Human infection is acquired through contact with infected animals. The human disease is a febrile disease with haemorrhages in severe cases: some patients have developed retinitis.

Virology

The following are some properties of the main arbovirus groups:

Togaviruses

1. More than 80 serological types—25 alphaviruses, more than 60 flaviviruses
2. RNA viruses
3. Roughly spherical, enveloped particles most are between 40 and 70 nm (Fig. 8.1)

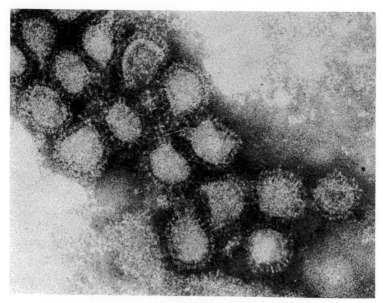

Fig 8.1 Togavirus. This photograph of sindbis virus shows roughly spherical particles with cubic symmetry and a surface fringe. × 200 000. (Photograph by Prof. C.R. Madeley.)

4. Most haemogglutinate avian erythrocytes, e.g. from day-old chicks or geese
5. Pathogenic for suckling mice
6. Grow in tissue culture.

Note: rubella virus is now classified as a togavirus but is not arthropod-borne.

Bunyavirus

1. More than 200 serological types, subdivided into bunyavirus, nairovirus, phlebovirus and uukuvirus
2. RNA viruses with single-stranded genome divided into three segments.
3. Roughly spherical particles 90–100 nm.
4. Some grow in cell culture.
5. Pathogenic for sucking mice.

Orbivirus

1. Classed as reoviruses, subdivided into 10 serological groups.
2. RNA viruses. Double-stranded genome in 10 segments.
3. Roughly spherical particles, 75–85 nm with inner nucleocapsid surrounded by outer, diffuse layer.
4. Grow in cell culture.

Diagnosis of arbovirus infection

Complex, requires facilities of specialist, reference laboratories.
    Generally by
1. *Serology* (complement fixation, haemagglutination-inhibition, neutralisation.)
2. *Isolation* from blood (e.g. throat swab, CSF etc) by inoculation of:
    (i) suckling mice
    (ii) cell culture (where appropriate)

Vaccine

The only widely used vaccine available for arboviruses is against yellow fever:

Yellow fever vaccine

Contains live attenuated virus of a strain known as 17D attenuated by repeated passage in chick embryos.

Prepared in chick embryos

Administered in one dose by subcutaneous injection.

Protection conferred is good, solid immunity which lasts for at least 10 years.

Safety: good, singularly free from side-effects.

9

Rabies, non-arthropod-borne haemorrhagic fevers, arenavirus infections

The diseases to be described in this chapter are zoonoses, i.e. they are acquired from animals which are reservoirs of infection. But note the reservoirs of Marburg and Ebola viruses have never been found.

RABIES

Rabies is a lethal form of encephalitis due to a virus which affects a wide variety of animal species: rabies is transmitted to man via the bite of an infected animal which is usually—but not always—a dog.

Clinical features

The incubation period is long—usually from 4 to 12 weeks but sometimes much longer; if the wound is on the head or neck the incubation period is shorter than for wounds on the limbs.

Virus spread from the wound to the CNS is via the nerves.

Symptoms: mainly of excitement, with tremor, muscular contractions and convulsions; typically spasm of the muscles of swallowing (hence the older name for the disease of 'hydrophobia' or fear of water) and increased sensitivity of the sensory nervous system—the classical syndrome of 'furious' rabies. Virus is present in saliva, skin and eyes as well as the brain.

Prognosis: the disease is virtually always fatal (although there have been rare reports of recovery); death often follows a convulsion. A rarer type is 'dumb' rabies seen in the West Indies and Central and South America: there is no hydrophobia and the course of illness is longer: this takes the form of an *ascending myelitis with paralysis* and is spread by the bite of infected vampire bats.

Pathology: despite the severity of the clinical disease, lesions in the CNS are often minimal with little evidence of destructive effects on cells; the main changes are the typical intracytoplasmic inclusions within neurones known as Negri bodies.

Epidemiology

Rabies is a natural infection of dogs, cats, bats and carnivorous wild animals such as foxes, wolves, skunks: infection is also found in rodents and cattle (especially in South America where the virus is spread by the bite of infected vampire bats). At present, in Europe, human exposure to rabies is generally more common from cats than dogs—except in Turkey where dog rabies is a particular problem. In underdeveloped countries, infection in urban dogs poses the main risk to man.

Virus is present in the saliva of infected animals—sometimes for up to four days before the onset of symptoms of the disease; animals which remain healthy for ten days after biting can be regarded as being free of virus at the time of biting.

Incidence of rabies after biting: relatively few—about 15%—of people bitten by a rabid animal develop the disease; rabies is more common after bites on the head or neck than after wounds on the limbs.

Britain is at present free from indigenous rabies. Rabies used to be present in animals in Britain but was eradicated by 1921; the strict six-month quarantine laws for animals imported into Britain have been successful in keeping out the disease. Smuggling of pet animals into Britain to avoid the quarantine regulations is fairly common and represents a potential source of importation of the virus. The main danger is that rabies might become established as a reservoir of infection in wild animals. If this happens, given Britain's fairly large fox population, it might prove difficult to eradicate the disease. Rabies is present in wild animals in all continents of the world with the exception of Australia (and Antartica). Most important from a British point of view is its spread as an epizootic, slowly moving westwards from Eastern Europe across Northern France to the area around the Channel ports.

Case to case spread: human patients are not a source of infection (despite the presence of virus in saliva).

Corneal transplant: cases of rabies in recipients of corneas from donors with undiagnosed rabies have been reported.

Virology

1. *A lyssavirus* within the *rhabdovirus* family: rabies is the most neurotropic of the antigenically related group of lyssaviruses which naturally infect many different animal species.
2. RNA virus.
3. Bullet-shaped, enveloped particles containing helically-coiled nucleoprotein; length 180 nm, diameter 70 to 80 nm (Fig. 9.1).
4. Haemagglutinates goose erythrocytes.
5. Grows in hamster kidney and chick embryo cell tissue cultures with eosinophilic cytoplasmic inclusions but usually without CPE.
6. Pathogenic for mice and other laboratory animals.

Diagnosis

Direct demonstration of virus

Specimens: hair-bearing skin (e.g. back of neck), corneal impression smears, brain tissue.

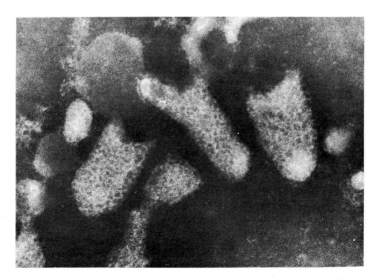

Fig. 9.1 Rabies virus. The nucleocapsid of the bullet-shaped particles has helical symmetry and is surrounded by an envelope. × 180 000. (Photograph by Prof. C R Madeley.)

Examine: for presence of rabies virus antigen by immunofluorescence.

Negri bodies: a less sensitive method of diagnosis: examine brain smears of the Ammon's horn of the hippocampus stained with Seller's stain for red intracytoplasmic inclusions (Negri bodies.)

Isolation

Specimens: brain tissue, saliva, CSF, urine.

Inoculate: mice intra-cerebrally.

Observe; For paralysis, convulsions; *post-mortem* for immunofluorescence with rabies antiserum and Negri bodies in brain cells.

Note: If rabies is suspected in a dog it should be kept under observation to see if the disease develops, and not killed right away; if it is killed before death due to the disease, Negri bodies may not have developed in sufficient numbers to be detected in histological sections. After death, the dog's head is sent to a specialist laboratory for examination.

Vaccination

Rabies vaccine was first developed by Pasteur in 1885; it consisted of virus attenuated by drying the spinal cords of infected rabbits for varying lenghts of time over KOH. Wild rabies virus is known as 'street' virus and attenuated virus as 'fixed' virus. All vaccines prepared for human use contain inactivated virus.

The long incubation period makes rabies a suitable disease for prophylactic immunisation after exposure.

After exposure—or suspicion of exposure—to rabies, the wound should be thoroughly washed with soap and water, alcohol, iodine solutions or quarternary ammonium compound; patients should then be given combined passive and active immunisation.

Passive immunisation: by injection of human anti-rabies immunoglobulin.
Active immunisation: should be started immediately after passive immunisation.

The main vaccines in use are:
Human diploid cell vaccine—now the vaccine of choice.

Contains: inactivated virus disrupted into subunits.

Prepared: in WI 38 human embryo lung cells.

Administered: intramuscularly or subcutaneously in 6 doses spaced at 0, 3, 7, 14, 30 and 90 days.

Protection: apparently effective; produces high levels of neutralizing antibody.

Safety: Good: does not cause neuroparalytic complications.

Semple vaccine—the successor to the original Pasteur vaccine and still in use in Africa and the Far East despite the risk of severe side effects (see below)

Contains: virus inactivated by phenol.

Prepared: from infected rabbit brain tissue.

Administered: subcutaneously in 21 daily injections with later booster doses

Protection: apparently effective.

Safety: severe neuroparalytic accidents due to allergic encephalomyelitis sometimes follow immunisation due to the repeated injections of nervous tissue.

Suckling mouse brain vaccine is used in Latin America: it has shown a lower incidence of neurological side-effects.

Duck embryo vaccine less used now: reduced risk of neurological side-effects.

Animal vaccines: live virus vaccines

Contain: live attenuated virus—HEP (high egg passage) Flury strain, SAD (Street Alabama Dufferin strain) or Kissling strain.

Used: for immunization of dogs, cats, cattle, etc.

Pre-exposure vaccination

Veterinary surgeons, animal handlers, laboratory workers or others at high risk from rabies should be given three doses of diploid cell vaccine one month apart with a booster dose 2 years later; two booster doses should be given if they are exposed to infection.

MARBURG AND EBOLA VIRUS DISEASES

Marburg is an exceptionally severe disease which appeared in 1967 as a single outbreak initially involving laboratory workers in Marburg, Frankfurt and Belgrade. The patients had handled tissues from the same batch of African green monkeys. Later, there were other cases in contacts of the patients. The monkeys were almost certainly infected during transit. Ebola appeared in Africa in 1976.

Clinical features

Clinically, the diseases are very severe, febrile illnesses with headache, myalgia, a maculo-papular rash and haemorrhagic manifestations; other features are vomiting, diarrhoea, hepatitis, pharyngitis and signs of renal and CNS involvement. There is leucopenia with atypical lymphocytes and plasma cells in the blood. *The case fatality rate is high*—considerably more than 50% in the Ebola outbreaks.

Infectiousness: a feature of both diseases is ability to spread directly from case to case: several of the infections have been in medical attendants of patients with the disease.

Epidemiology

Marburg disease appeared again in 1975 in two young people in South Africa. In 1976 there were severe outbreaks of a similar disease with many deaths in Sudan and Zaire. These outbreaks were due to a morphologically similar but antigenically different virus now named Ebola virus (after the river in the epidemic area in Zaire). The reservoirs of the viruses—almost certainly some species of wild animal—have not been identified.

Virology

1. Unclassified—perhaps a new family, filoviruses
2. RNA viruses
3. Unusual virus particles, long, filamentous, with the ends bent or branching. Variable length, diameter 80 nm. Particles have surface spikes.
4. Grow in various tissue cultures without CPE but with intra-cytoplasmic inclusions
5. Pathogenic for guinea-pigs, monkeys and other laboratory animals.

Diagnosis

The diseases have a very characteristic clinical picture. Confirmation of the virus aetiology in the original outbreak was obtained by isolating the virus in laboratory animals.

Isolation

Specimen: blood

Inoculate: guinea pigs or cell cultures

Observe:
1. *guinea pigs* for signs of febrile illness with detection of virus antigen by immunofluorescence in lesions in liver, lymph nodes or spleen.
2. *cell cultures* for intracytoplasmic inclusions by immunofluorescence.

Serology
Complement fixation test.

ARENAVIRUSES

There are four human pathogenic arenaviruses:
1. Lymphocytic choriomeningitis
2. Lassa fever virus
3. Junin virus
4. Macrhpo virus

The natural hosts of all four viruses are mice or rats. Infection is acquired by inhalation or ingestion of materials contaminated with rodent excreta. But Lassa fever can be acquired by direct contact with a case of the disease.

LYMPHOCYTIC CHORIOMENINGITIS

The virus causes widespread natural infection in mice and is excreted in the urine and faeces of infected mice; transmission to man appears to be a rare event. The disease has also been acquired from pet and laboratory hamsters.

The disease is of interest from an immunological point of view since mice are not uncommonly infected in utero; when this happens they have a generalised infection with high titres of virus in all tissues and organs; however the mice remain symptomless although they later succumb to glomerulonephritis due to immune complex deposition in kidneys.

Clinical features

The most important syndrome in man is aseptic meningitis; sometimes meningo-encephalitis is seen; the virus also causes an influenza-like febrile illness.

LASSA FEVER

A serious febrile disease endemic in West Africa which was first reported in Lassa in Nigeria. The virus is highly infectious and spreads readily by contact—including to medical and nursing personnel looking after patients. Rats are the reservoir of the virus.

Clinical features

The illness is severe with fever, vomiting, cough, weakness and malaise; sore throat with ulcers in the mouth and pharynx and cervical lymphadenopathy are characteristic features; abdominal pain, myalgia with diarrhoea and headache are common and the blood count shows leucopenia; the case fatality is high—around a third of patients in reported outbreaks have died.

ARGENTINIAN AND BOLIVIAN HAEMORRHAGIC FEVERS

Due to Junin and Machupo viruses respectively. Clinically both are severe diseases with haemorrhage and renal, cardiovascular and sometimes neurological symptoms. The reservoirs of both viruses are mouse-like rodents. The Argentinian disease is rural and spreads mainly during the maize harvest from mice which inhabit the maize fields. The Bolivian disease is mostly acquired in houses.

Virology

1. Arenas are a large family of viruses
2. RNA viruses—the genome consists of two unique (i.e. not identical) virus specific RNA segments but the particle also contains host cell RNA species (see below).
3. Medium-sized, 110 nm enveloped particles with internal granules which are host cell ribosomes associated with the different host cell RNAs.
4. Grow in cell culture.
5. Pathogenic for mice and guinea-pigs.

Diagnosis

Serology
Complement fixation text (lymphocytic choriomeningitis) Immunofluorescence (Lassa fever)

Isolation

Specimen: blood, throat swabs, CSF etc.

Inoculate:
1. (for lymphocytic choriomeningitis) mice intracerebrally: observe for spasm of hind legs, tremors, convulsions and death.
2. (for Lassa fever) Vero cell cultures: observe for CPE—or possibly virus antigen by immunofluorescence.

HAEMORRHAGIC FEVER WITH RENAL SYNDROME (HFRS)

Originally called Korean haemorrhagic fever and first described in U.S. soldiers in the Korean war. Now seen in two epidemic forms:
1. *Far East*: severe febrile illness with haemorrhage
2. *Scandinavia and Eastern Europe*: milder haemorrhagic fever with renal involvement; known as nephropathia epidemica.

Cause: Haantaan virus—a bunyavirus.

Epidemiology

A natural infection of mice—probably worldwide. Although mostly reported in epidemic form as described above, there have been occasional infections in other countries—including Britain. Some cases in Belgium were traced to infection in laboratory mice.

Diagnosis

Serology: by immunofluorescence

10

Herpesvirus diseases

There are a large number of herpesviruses. Most animal species, including man, are hosts for a particular herpes virus and sometimes two or more viruses. All are morphologically identical and have the important property of remaining *latent*, in potentially viable form, within the cells of the host after primary infection. Latent virus persists for long periods of time—probably throughout life: some herpesviruses reactivate from time to time from the latent state to produce recurrent infection.

There are four human herpesviruses:
1. Herpes simplex virus
2. Varicella-zoster virus
3. Cytomegalovirus
4. Epstein-Barr virus.

HERPES SIMPLEX VIRUS

Herpes simplex virus is unusual among viruses in causing a wide variety of clinical syndromes: the basic lesions are vesicles but these can take many different forms.

Clinical features

Diseases due to the virus are in two categories:
Primary: when the virus is first encountered.
Reactivation: recurrent infections due to reactivation of latent virus.

Primary infections

Virtually everyone becomes infected with the virus but most primary infections are symptomless. Below are listed the main clinical manifestations when primary infection is accompanied by symptoms.

1. *Gingivo-stomatitis*: vesicles inside the mouth on the buccal mucosa and on the gums: these ulcerate and become coated with a greyish slough. Although this is the commonest primary disease, because kissing is the main route of virus spread, vesicles may be produced at other sites, most often on the head or neck.

2. *Herpetic whitlow*: due to implantation of the virus into the fingers: the lesion produced is very similar to a staphylococcal whitlow but the exudate is serous rather than purulent: an occupational hazard of doctors and nurses especially in anaesthetists or neurosurgical nurses, who deal with unconscious patients who are intubated: infection is acquired through contamination of the hands by virus in saliva or respiratory secretions.

3. *Conjunctivitis and keratitis*: primary herpes can involve the eye—and both conjunctiva and cornea: the eyelids are usually swollen and there are often vesicles and ulcers on them.

4. *Kaposi's varicelliform eruption* is a superinfection of eczematous skin: mainly seen in young children, it can be a serious disease with a significant case fatality rate.

5. *Acute necrotising encephalitis*: herpes encephalitis is a very rare but extremely severe disease: clinically, it presents with the sudden onset of fever, mental confusion and headache: the main site of infection is the temporal lobe where the disease causes necrosis. Recently a milder form of herpes encephalitis with a better prognosis has been described—usually in children. It is uncertain if herpes encephalitis is a primary infection or a reactivation.

6. *Genital herpes*: a vesicular eruption of the genital area most often due to a variant of the virus known as herpes simplex virus type 2: type 2 virus is antigenically and biologically slightly different (although also similar in many properties) to the more common type 1 herpes simplex virus which infects the head and neck; genital herpes is usually sexually transmitted. But note, genital herpes is due to type 1 virus in from a quarter to a third of cases.

7. *Neonatal infection*: severe generalised infection in neonates is usually acquired from a primary genital infection in the mother when no maternal antibody is present for the protection of the child: affected infants have jaundice, hepatosplenomegaly, thrombocytopaenia and large vesicular lesions on the skin: there is a high case fatality rate: usually due to herpes simplex virus type 2.

8. *Generalised infection* in adults is a rare manifestation of primary infection with type 1 virus: *herpes hepatitis* has also been described.

Latency

During primary infection, the virus travels from the site of infection in the mouth to the trigeminal—and probably other cranial and cervical ganglia also. The mode of travel is unknown but is probably via the nerves. Virus remains in the ganglia in a potentially viable state and in a proportion of people, *reactivates to cause recurrent infection*. Even in the absence of recurrent infection virus can be isolated from the trigeminal ganglia in most normal people. The state of the virus in the ganglion cells is unknown but it is almost certainly not present as intact virions: the most popular theory is that latent virus is in the form of virus DNA integrated into the cellular chromosomes. In genital herpes, type 2 virus becomes latent in the sacral ganglia.

Reactivation of virus is provoked by various stimuli including common colds, sunlight (possibly a result of exposure to ultra-violet light), pneumonia, stress, menstruation, etc. Reactivation recurs sporadically, sometimes often, throughout life.

Neutralising antibody is formed after primary infection but— surprisingly—does not prevent reactivation: this may be because the virus is protected from serum antibody as it travels within the axons of sensory nerves to the site of recurrent infection. Reactivation does not stimulate a rise in titre of herpes antibody.

Clinical manifestations of reactivation:

1. *Cold sores*: or vesicles round mucocutaneous junctions of nose and mouth are the most common: the vesicles progress to pustules with crust formation: the virus travels down the maxillary or mandibular branches of the trigeminal nerve to reach areas of the skin supplied by these nerves; herpetic vesicles can recur—but more rarely—at other sites on the skin: genital lesions also recur and these are mainly due to type 2 virus.
2. *Keratitis*: reactivation less commonly affects the eye: recurrent lesions are usually restricted to the cornea and the conjunctiva is not involved: virus reaches the cornea via the ophthalmic

branch of the trigeminal nerve: lesions take the form of a branching or *dendritic ulcer*: if recurrence is frequent, scarring develops and in a few cases the disease progresses to a severe, destructive uveitis.

3. *Immunosuppressive therapy*: especially in renal transplant patients is sometimes associated with severe, extensive cold sores; usually in the mouth, these may be necrotic and spread to involve large areas of the face and into the oesophagus.

Epidemiology

Infectivity: herpes simplex is not a very infectious virus and there are, for example, no outbreaks of herpes infections in the community.

Spread: by close personal contact, e.g. kissing (type 1 virus), sexual intercourse (type 2 virus).

Sources: generally people with herpetic lesions; however, carriers of the latent virus from time to time secrete virus in their saliva without any symptoms and this may act as a source of (undetected) infection.

Age: infection is most common in childhood and is usually symptomless: there is another peak in incidence during adolescence due to kissing as contact with the opposite sex increases.

Infection: is virtually universal in human populations and in elderly people the incidence of antibody (indicating previous infection) is almost 100 per cent.

Virology

1. Roughly spherical particle with cubic symmetry, medium size—100 nm, with 162 projecting hollow-cored capsomeres; many of the particles are surrounded by a loose envelope of material partially derived from the host cell (Fig. 10.1).
2. Double-stranded DNA.
3. Two types of virus—1 and 2: types 1 and 2 share antigens in common (group-specific) but possess type-specific antigens also: although their DNA shows some homology, the two types of DNA can be readily distinguished by restriction enzyme

analysis. Virus-specified proteins of the two viruses are produced in approximately equal numbers but can be distinguished by differences in their molecular weights when separated by electrophoresis in polyacrylamide gels.

4. Grows in various tissue cultures with characteristic CPE with ballooning and rounding of cells.

5. Grows on chorio-allantoic membrane with production of tiny white pocks.

6. Pathogenic for laboratory animals causing encephalitis.

Diagnosis

Isolation

Specimens: vesicle fluid, skin swab, saliva, conjunctival fluid, corneal scrapings, brain biopsy.

Inoculate: cell cultures, e.g. BHK21 (a hamster kidney cell line), human embryo lung cells.

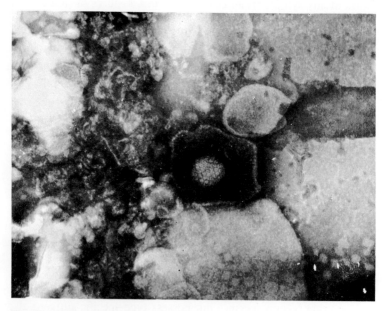

Fig. 10.1 Herpes simplex virus. The particle has cubic symmetry and the capsid is composed of hollow-cored capsomeres. There is a loose, baggy envelope. × 108 000. (Photograph by Dr E.A.C. Follett.)

Observe: for CPE of rounded cells.

Type: by neutralisation test with standard antiserum; immuno-fluorescence

Serology

Complement fixation test, useful for diagnosing primary infections; difficult to interpret in recurrent infections because of high levels of existing antibody and because recurrences usually do not cause a rise in titre.

Chemotherapy (see also Chapter 14)

Acyclovir: treatment of herpes simplex has been revolutionised by the introduction of this non-toxic drug which has a specific inhibitory action on herpes simplex virus replication.

Administered: intravenously (best), orally or topically

Indications: herpes encephalitis, severe or generalized herpes
(given systemically)
genital herpes (systemically or orally)
dendritic ulcers, cold sores, possibly genital herpes (topically)
prophylaxis in immunocompromised patients.
Idoxuridine (0.1% solution): still regularly used topically in the treatment of herpes keratitis. Herpetic skin lesions and whitlows can be treated topically with stronger solutons (i.e. 5%—or 40% for whitlows—in dimethyl sulphoxide).

VARICELLA-ZOSTER VIRUS

Varicella (chickenpox) and zoster (shingles—but also sometimes called 'herpes zoster') are different diseases due to the same virus.
Varicella is the primary illness.
Zoster is a recurrent manifestation of infection.

VARICELLA

Clinical features

Varicella—a common childhood fever. There is a mild febrile illness with a characteristic vesicular rash; vesicles appear in successive waves so that lesions of different age are present together; the vesicles (in which there are giant cells) develop into pustules.

Complications are rare: post-infectious encephalomyelitis, haemorrhagic (fulminating) varicella; in adults pneumonia is a relatively common and serious complication and may be followed by permanent pulmonary calcification.

Congenital varicella: exceedingly rare: maternal varicella in early pregnancy is occasionally followed by a syndrome in the infant of limb hypoplasia, muscular atrophy and cerebral and psychomotor retardation.

Perinatal or neonatal varicella: maternal varicella near the time of delivery may also affect the child: if the mother contracts varicella more than 5 days before delivery, the disease in the child is usually mild: this is because the child's disease is modified by placentally-transmitted early maternal antibody: when maternal varicella is contracted within 5 days of delivery, there is not time for maternal antibody to be produced and cross the placenta, and the child is liable to develop severe disease.

Immunity: attack is followed by solid and long lasting immunity to varicella—but *not to zoster*.

Epidemiology

Seasonal distribution: highest incidence is in autumn and winter.

Spread: via nose and mouth by droplet infection from infectious saliva; virus is also present in skin lesions.

Varicella is an epidemic contagious disease; it may be acquired by contact with cases either of varicella or (less commonly) of zoster.

Zoster

Due to reactivation of virus latent in dorsal root or cranial nerve ganglia following—and usually many years after—childhood varicella.

Mainly affects adults: clinically there is an eruption of *painful vesicles* in areas of skin corresponding in distribution to one or more sensory nerves; the most commonly affected are the thoracic nerves, less often the cranial—notably the ophthalmic—nerves.

When *dorsal root ganglia* are involved there is a segmental rash which extends from the middle of the back in a horizontal strip round the side of the chest wall—'a belt of roses from hell'.

When *the ophthalmic nerve of the trigeminal ganglion* is affected the rash is distributed within the skin supplied by that nerve depending on the roots affected. This may cause a sharply demarcated area of lesions down one side of the forehead and scalp: in about half the patients, there are lesions in the eye.

Ramsay Hunt syndrome is a rare form of zoster: the eruption is on the tympanic membrane and the external auditory canal and there is often a facial nerve palsy.

Residual neuralgia—which may be severe—often follows zoster in the elderly.

Neurological signs are sometimes seen, e.g. paralysis.

Note: Virus is present in both the skin lesions and in the corresponding dorsal root ganglion.

Epidemiology

Zoster—unlike varicella—is not acquired by contact with cases of either varicella or zoster—although it may give rise to cases of varicella in susceptible contacts.
Cases are *sporadic* there is *no seasonal distribution*.

Virology

1. One serological type; in the electron microscope the particle is that of a typical herpes virus and is morphologically identical to that of herpes simplex.
2. Grows slowly in tissue cultures of human cells (e.g. human embryo lung) with focal CPE but *the virus remains cell associated*, i.e. no free virus is released into the medium.

Diagnosis

Serology. Complement fixation test: unlike reactivations of herpes simplex, zoster usually causes a rise in antibody titre.

Direct demonstration of typical herpes virus particles in vesicle fluid by electron microscopy is a quick method of confirming a clinical diagnosis (but note, this does not distinguish varicella-zoster from herpes simplex virus).

Isolation. Rarely attempted.

Treatment

Severe varicella or zoster (e.g. in the immunocompromised) can be treated with intravenous acyclovir: the virus is less sensitive than herpes simplex.

CYTOMEGALOVIRUS

Cytomegalovirus diseases are examples of *'opportunistic infections'*, i.e. the virus rarely causes disease unless precipitating factors are present which lower the normal resitance of the host. Like rubella, cytomegalovirus can infect the fetus during maternal infection in pregnancy.

Symptomless infections are common: about 50% of the adult population has antibody to the virus almost always without developing any symptoms of disease.

Latency: the virus is known to reactivate from the latent state, the site is uncertain but is probably polymorphonuclear leucocytes or lymphocytes.

There are two types of disease due to cytomegalovirus:
1. Congenital

A more difficult problem than congenital rubella because:
1. Maternal infection is almost always symptomless
2. The fetus can be damaged by infection in any of the three trimesters of pregnancy.
3. Fetal infection can follow reactivation as well as primary maternal infection.
4. Approximately 0.4% of British children are congenitally infected but most do not suffer sequelae (termination therefore presents ethical problems).

Clinical features

The majority of congenitally infected neonates show no signs or symptoms and diagnosis is made by virological tests. Many of these children develop normally but some show neurological sequelae later in life principally:
1. deafness
2. mental retardation
About a fifth of infected children show clinical signs of infection and in a few cases this takes the form of the severe generalised— or cytomegalic inclusion—disease.

Severe generalised infection (Cytomegalic inclusion disease)

Signs and symptoms: affected infants have jaundice, hepatosplenomegaly, blood dyscrasias such as thrombocytopenia and haemolytic anaemia; the brain is almost always inv ʳed with microcephaly and motor disorders; surviving infants are usually deaf and mentally retarded. Cytomegalovirus is probably the cause of about 10% of cases of microcephaly.

Affected organs: show characteristic enlarged cells (hence the prefix 'cytomegalo') with large intranuclear 'owl's eye' inclusions. Although this form of congenital cytomegalovirus infection is relatively rare, the effects are so severe that the disease represents a considerable medical and social problem.

2. Postnatal

Hepatitis

In children, cytomegalovirus causes hepatitis with enlargement of the liver and disturbance of liver function tests; jaundice may or may not be present.

Infectious mononucleosis

In adults, infection may take the form of an illness like infectious mononucleosis (see below) but with a negative Paul Bunnell reaction and no lymphadenopathy or pharyngitis. There is fever, hepatitis and lymphocytosis with atypical lymphocytes in the peripheral blood; the syndrome is sometimes seen after transfusion with fresh unfrozen blood—presumably cytomegalovirus, which may occasionally be present in the donor's blood, is normally inactivated by storage at 4°C.

Infection in the immunocompromised

Disseminated infection is sometimes seen when immunosuppressive therapy or severe debilitating disease, such as neoplasm is present to lower the host's resistance. There are usually widespread lesions involving lungs as well as other organs and tissues, e.g. adrenals, liver and alimentary tract. This is a major complication of transplantation surgery:

Renal transplant patients are subject to frequent infections with cytomegalovirus—probably mainly reactivations of latent virus—but these are not always associated with signs or symptoms of disease. *Pneumonitis* and, rarely, *retinitis* due to cytomegalovirus have been reported in transplant patients.

Bone marrow transplant patients are even more susceptible than those with renal grafts (possibly due to the greater immunosuppression with the former patients). Cytomegalovirus pneumonitis is an important cause of death in them.

Virology

1. Electron microscopy—a typical herpes virus particle.
2. Grows slowly in cultures of human embryo lung cells with characteristic focal CPE and intranuclear 'owl's eye' inclusions.

Diagnosis

Isolation

Specimens: urine, throat swab.

Inoculate: human embryo lung cell cultures.

Observe: for characteristic CPE of foci of swollen cells; this may take from 2 to 3 weeks to appear.

Serology

Immunofluorescence, ELISA tests for IgM, complement fixation test.

Demonstration

Of typical intranuclear 'owl's eye' inclusion in cells of urinary sediment or other tissues.

EPSTEIN-BARR (EB) VIRUS

Epstein-Barr virus is named after the virologists who first observed it when examining cultures of lymphoblasts from Burkitt's lymphoma in the electron microscope.

EB virus infection is widespread in human populations and most people have antibody to it by the time they reach adulthood.

Most infections are symptomless: especially if acquired during childhood; if infection is delayed until adult life there is greater likelihood of disease; this takes the form of *infectious mononucleosis* or glandular fever.

Persistence of virus: EB virus persists in latent form within lymphocytes following primary infection: the virus is present in the form of viral DNA—both free in the cytoplasm and integrated into the cellular chromosone.

Burkitt's lymphoma: the virus may cause this cancer of the lymphoid tissues which is common in African children (see Chapter 16).

INFECTIOUS MONONUCLEOSIS (glandular fever)

Clinical features

Incubation period: is long—from 4 to 7 weeks.

Route of infection: close or intimate contact, e.g. kissing; the virus has been demonstrated in cells in salivary secretions. The disease is most prevalent amongst young adults, especially student populations (of whom a sizeable minority have no antibody).

Signs and symptoms: low-grade fever with generalized lymphadenopathy and sore throat due to exudative tonsillitis; malaise, anorexia and tiredness to a severe degree are characteristic features; splenomegaly is common and most cases have abnormal liver function tests; a proportion have palpable enlargement of the liver and frank jaundice is not uncommon.

Mononucleosis: or—more correctly—a relative and absolute lymphocytosis is a diagnostic feature; at least 10% and usually more of the lymphocytes are atypical with enlarged misshapen nuclei and more cytoplasm than normal; the atypical lymphocytes are both B and T cells.

Paul Bunnell test: infectious mononucleosis is characteristically associated with the appearance in the blood of heterophil antibody to sheep erythrocytes; this antibody can be removed by absorption with ox erythrocytes but not by absorption with guinea pig kidney. The differential absorption and the haemagglutination test with sheep erythrocytes constitute the Paul Bunnell test which is diagnostic of infectious mononucleosis: development of other non-specific antibodies (e.g. rheumatoid factor and anti-i cold agglutinin) are also features of the disease.

EB virus antibody: is produced during infection but antibody usually is present before symptoms develop; the presence of EB virus-specific IgM is a useful confirmatory diagnostic test.

Duration: in most cases of infectious mononucleosis symptoms last from 2 to 3 weeks but, in a proportion, the illness may persist for weeks or even months.

Virology

1. Electron microscopy—a typical herpesvirus
2. Grows in suspension cultures of human lymphoblasts.
3. EB virus can be detected or isolated by its ability to 'transform' normal human lymphocytes into a continuously dividing line of cells.

Diagnosis

Serology

1. Paul Dunnell test.
2. Demonstration of EB virus-specific IgM by immunofluorescence; the antibody tested is that directed against the viral capsid antigen.

Haematology

Demonstration of atypical lymphocytes in the peripheral blood.

11

Mumps, measles, rubella

Mumps, measles and rubella are, with varicella, the common childhood fevers. Measles has been, at least partially, controlled by vaccination and this has altered its traditional epidemiology. Rubella vaccination is aimed at protecting against the risk of fetal infection while not interfering with naturally-acquired immunity. An effective mumps vaccine is available but is not in general use.

MUMPS

Clinical features

Incubation period: relatively long—18 to 21 days.

Clinically: classical mumps is a febrile illness with inflammation of salivary glands causing characteristitic swelling of parotid and submaxillary glands.

Aseptic meningitis: (less often meningoencephalitis) are frequent neurological complications of mumps; occasionally there is muscular weakness or paralysis. Mumps meningitis is not accompanied by parotitis in 50% of cases. *Nerve deafness* is a rare complication.

Other complications: *orchitis*, *pancreatitis* and—very rarely—*oophoritis* and *thyroiditis* are seen in association with mumps; about 20% of adult males who contract mumps develop orchitis.

Immunity: an attack is followed by solid and long-lasting immunity; second attacks are very rare.

Mumps is a generalised infection by a virus with a predilection for the CNS (neurotropism) and for glandular tissue.

Epidemiology

Spread is by droplet infection with infectious respiratory secretions.

Seasonal incidence: highest in the spring.

Age distribution: most frequent in children aged from 5 to 15 years but not uncommon in young adults: outbreaks have been reported in recruit populations.

Infectiousness: lower than measles; as a result infection in childhood is not as common as with measles and a significant proportion of adults are non-immune.

Important because of the relative frequency of neurological complications especially when mumps infects adults; mumps is an important cause of aseptic meningitis.

Epidemics of mumps last about 2 years and are followed by a year when the incidence of infection is low; another period of high incidence then appears.

Virology

1. Paramyxovirus, one serological type
2. RNA virus
3. Enveloped particles, rather large in size—110 to 170 nm; helical symmetry
4. Haemagglutinates fowl erythrocytes
5. Grows in amniotic cavity of chick embryo and in monkey kidney and other tissue cultures with haemadsorption.

Diagnosis

Serology (widely used)
Complement fixation test: Two antigens are used:
1. 'S' or soluble antigen (the nucleoprotein core of the virus particle);
2. 'V' or viral antigen (found on the surface of the virus particle). Antibody to 'S' antigen tends to diminish sooner than antibody to 'V' antigen; it can therefore be a useful indicator of recent infection.
'V' antibody usually persists for years.

Isolation (mainly used for diagnosis of mumps meningitis)

Specimens: CSF, possibly throat washings.

Inoculate: monkey kidney tissue cultures

Observe: for haemadsorption of fowl erythrocytes;

Identify virus: by inhibition of haemadsorption or haemagglutination with standard antiserum.

Vaccine

A mumps vaccine has recently become available although not widely used in Britain, it is popular in USA

Contains: live attenuated virus grown in chick embryo cells.

Administered: in one dose subcutaneously.

Protection: apparently good.

Reactions: occasionally mild fever.

MEASLES

Clinical features

Measles is the most common of the childhood fevers; in uncomplicated cases it is a mild disease but complications are relatively frequent.

Prodromal symptoms are respiratory e.g. nasal discharge and suffusion of the eyes.

The main illness of measles follows; fever—which may be high—with a maculopapular rash lasting from two to five days: the rash is an enanthem (as well as an exanthem) and characteristic spots (Koplik's spots) appear in the buccal mucosa inside the cheek and mouth.

Immunity following measles is life-long: but note, measles itself has a suppressive effect on the immune system.

Complications

1. Respiratory
2. Neurological

1. *Respiratory infections*: are the most common and are seen in about 4% of patients; these include bronchitis, bronchiolitis, croup and bronchopneumonia; *otitis media* is also seen in about 2.5% of cases. Before the advent of the antibiotics these infections were more frequent and were largely responsible for the mortality associated with measles.

Giant cell pneumonia: a rare complication, seen mainly in children immunodeficient or with chronic debilitating diseases; due to direct invasion of the lungs by measles virus and usually fatal: there are numerous multinucleated giant cells in the lungs at post-mortem.

2. *Neurological complications*:

Two types of encephalitis are seen:

(i) *Encephalitis or post-infectious encephalomyelitis*: a serious condition which follows measles in about one in every 1000 cases; the mortality rate is about 50% and many survivors have residual neurological symptoms. Encephalitis commonly presents with drowsiness, vomiting, headache and convulsions.

(ii) *Subacute sclerosing panencephalitis*: A very rare but severe, chronic, neurological disease seen in children and young adults. The presenting symptoms are of personality and behavioural changes with intellectual impairment; the disease progresses to convulsions, myoclonic movements and increasing neurological deterioration leading to coma and death. Due to persistent infection with measles virus following primary and usually uncomplicated measles several years previously; affected children have high titres of measles antibody in their serum and both IgM and IgG measles-specific antibody in the CSF.

At post mortem, there are numerous intranuclear inclusions throughout the brain: measles virus has been grown from brain tissue.

Epidemiology

The attack rate in measles is high: virtually everybody in Britain under the age of 15 years has had the disease or—nowadays—been vaccinated against it. When the disease has been introduced into isolated communities where measles is not endemic and the entire population is susceptible, attack rates of more than 99% have been recorded.

Spread is by inhalation of respiratory secretions from patients in the early stages of the disease.

Epidemics: measles in Britain used to appear in epidemics every second year—probably because in two years sufficient new susceptible hosts had been born into the community for the virus to become epidemic again; in non-epidemic years, measles was endemic but the number of cases was lower than in epidemic years.

The introduction of measles vaccine has caused a marked reduction in the incidence both of measles and measles encephalitis.

In countries like Britain, where there is little poverty and malnutrition, measles is a mild disease with a low mortality rate.

In under-developed countries, e.g. West Africa, measles is a severe disease and a serious cause of death in childhood.

Virology

1. Paramyxovirus, one serological type
2. RNA virus
3. Enveloped particles, rather large size, 120 to 250 nm; helical symmetry
4. Haemagglutinates and haemolyses monkey erythrocytes
5. Grows in human amnion cells with syncytial CPE of multinucleated giant cells.

Diagnosis

Serology: complement fixation test: detection of measles IgM by immunofluorescence

Direct demonstration of viral antigen by immunofluorescence in nasopharyngeal aspirates.

Vaccine

Measles vaccination has been introduced to reduce the morbidity due to respiratory complications and the risk of encephalitis. Routine immunisation in the second year of life is officially recommended in Britain.

Contains: virus attenuated by passage in tissue cultures of chick embryo fibroblasts.

Administered: in one dose subcutaneously.

Protection: good: however, although the immunity conferred is, for the most part, long-lasting, cases of atypical measles have been reported in adolescents who had been vaccinated as children: this suggests that the immunity may not last so long as that following natural infection. It would be potentially serious if vaccination in childhood left some people unprotected in adult life when the natural disease is more severe.

Reactions: reactions such as fever and rash are fairly common but are milder than in natural measles.

Safety: vaccinated children are not infectious of others although virus multiplies in their bodies.

Normal immunoglobulin

Normal immunoglobulin is derived from pooled human sera and therefore contains measles antibody: it has been used to confer pasive immunity to infants and other unsually susceptible individuals who have been in contact with cases of measles.

RUBELLA

Rubella is a mild childhood fever but if infection is contracted in early pregnancy the virus can cause congenital abnormalities in the fetus.

Clinical features

A mild febrile illness with a macular rash which spreads down from the face and behind the ears; there is usually pharyngitis and enlargement of the cervical—and especially the posterior cervical—lymph glands.

Virus is present in both blood and pharyngeal secretions and is excreted during the incubation period for up to seven days before the appearance of the rash.

Many infections are symptomless.

Complications are rare: post-infectious encephalomyelitis, thrombocytopenic purpura and arthralgia or painful joints.

Epidemiology

Mainly attacks children under 15 years of age but a proportion reach adult life without being infected so that rubella in adults is not uncommon; about 15% of women of child-bearing age have not been infected and are therefore non-immune.

Infection is endemic in the community with epidemics every few years: the most extensive outbreak recorded was in the USA in 1964 when there were 1 800 000 cases.

The teratogenic properties of the virus were first discovered in Australia in 1941: Gregg (an ophthalmologist) noticed an increased number of cases of congenital cataract following an epidemic of rubella: affected infants had been born to mothers with a history of rubella in early pregnancy and he concluded that early maternal rubella could cause congenital defects in the offspring.

Congenital defects follow rubella only in the first 16 weeks of pregnancy; after that rubella does not damage the fetus.

The main defects are a triad of:

Cataract
Nerve deafness
Cardiac abnormalities (e.g. patent ductus arteriosus, ventricular septal defect, pulmonary artery stenosis, Fallot's tetralogy.)

The affected infants have various other disorders due to generalised infection which, together with the defects, are known as *the rubella syndrome*; these are:

Hepatosplenomegaly
Thrombocytopenic purpura
Low birth weight
Mental retardation
Jaundice
Anaemia
Lesions in the metaphyses of the long bones.

The incidence of defects after maternal rubella in the first three months of pregnancy has varied from 10% to 54% in different studies. Maternal rubella at this time also is associated with a higher proportion of abortions and stillbirths.

Time of infection: the severity and multiplicity of defects are increased when infection is in the earliest weeks of pregnancy.

The incidence of both deafness and defective vision further increases as congenitally-infected children grow up — probably due to easier recognition of these defects in older children.

Subacute sclerosing parencephalitis has been reported as a rare, late, complication of congenital rubella.

Infants with the rubella syndrome have IgM antibody to rubella virus and therefore are immunologically competent (the maternal antibody which crosses the placenta is IgG antibody).

Antibody protects against re-infection and second attacks appear to be rare (some reported second attacks may have been due to other virus infections misdiagnosed as rubella since rubella is not a particularly distinctive illness).

Virology

1. A non-arthropod-borne togavirus, one serological type.
2. RNA virus.
3. Pleomorphic-enveloped particles, medium size — 50 to 75 nm; helical symmetry.
4. Haemagglutinates bird erythrocytes, e.g. from day-old chicks.
5. Grows in a rabbit kidney cell line — RK 13 with production of CPE and in other tissue cultures but without CPE.

Diagnosis

Laboratory diagnosis is now widely used for confirmation of the diagnosis of rubella — usually in a pregnant woman or in suspected congenital rubella; also used to detect non-immune women who may be offered vaccination.

Serology

IgM antibody: recent infection with rubella virus is best diagnosed by the demonstration of IgM rubella antibody in a single sample of blood; most often detected by ELISA or by immunofluorescence with confirmation by fractionation of serum on a sucrose gradient: the fraction containing IgM antibodies is then tested by haemagglutination-inhibition.

Haemagglutination-inhibition test: quite a sensitive technique for detecting rubella antibody: active rubella (e.g. in pregnancy) can be diagnosed by demonstration of a rising titre of IgG. Specimens need only be 3 days apart.

Isolation: (most often used for the diagnosis of congenital rubella).

Inoculate: RK13 (rabbit kidney) or SIRC (rabbit cornea) cell lines.

Observe: for CPE

Single radial haemolysis: widely used for detecting immunity in pregnant women or in women at special risk e.g. children's nurses, schoolteachers: it does not measure antibody titre and is not suitable for the diagnosis of rubella.

Vaccination

Two live attenuated virus vaccines are in use in Britain:
1. RA 27/3
2. Cendehill

Contain: virus attenuated by passage in tissue culture; virus is grown in either primary rabbit kidney cells (Cendehill) or W138 human embryo fibroblasts (RA 27/3).

Administered: one dose subcutaneously.

Protection: good—rather better with RA 27/3 than Cendehill—immunity so far appears to be relatively long-lasting.

Reactions: mild; sometimes slight fever and rash; mild arthralgia is seen occasionally in adult females.

Viral excretion: Many vaccinees excrete virus from the nasopharynx but are apparently non-infectious to contacts.

Indications: schoolgirls aged 11 to 14 years; non-immune women of childbearing age, especially those at special risk e.g. nurses, schoolteachers, doctors: pregnancy must be avoided for three months after vaccination.

Contra-indication: Pregnant women should not be given vaccine since vaccine virus is capable of crossing the placenta to infect the fetus.

Note: rubella vaccination has been in force in Britain for fourteen years; but has been slow in achieving a reduction in the incidence of congenital rubella; the first schoolgirls who were vaccinated are now grown up and a protective effect has become apparent.

Passive immunisation with rubella-specific immunoglobulin may have some slight attenuating or prophylactic effect in rubella. It may be considered for use in maternal rubella if termination is refused.

PARVOVIRUS

A small, single-stranded DNA virus which causes *erythema infectiosum* which is also known as 'fifth disease' and 'slapped cheek syndrome'. Clinically this is a febrile disease in children, often epidemic, with a facial maculopapular rash causing flushed cheeks. In patients with erythrocyte abnormalities such as sickle cell anaemia and hereditary spherocytosis this virus can cause haemalytic crises, apparently by replicating in bone marrow cells to inhibit erythropoiesis.

Symptomless infection is common and around 30–40% of the population have antibodies of the virus.

First detected by *electron microscopy* in serum from patients, it does not grow in tissue culture.

Animal parvoviruses: also exist and epidemics of infection have been recorded in dogs and cats.

Diagnosis: serology radioimmune assay for IgM.

12

Poxvirus diseases

Most, possibly all, animal species are host to their own poxviruses. Man's was smallpox—one of the most fatal of all virus infections. Yet it was defeated—for three reasons:
1. Man was the only host animal
2. There was an effective vaccine against it (originally discovered by Jenner in 1796)
3. By the mid 20th century there were only a limited number of areas of endemic infection.

Eradication

In 1967 the World Health Organisation embarked on a Smallpox Eradication campaign. This was based on policy of 'search and containment' i.e. isolation of cases and the tracing and vaccination of contacts. There was continuing and long-term surveillance of previously endemic areas before these were declared smallpox-free. The main endemic areas were India, Pakistan and Bangladesh and, in Africa, Ethiopia and Somalia. The campaign was outstandingly successful and smallpox has now been eradicated: the World Health Organisation declared the world free from smallpox in May 1980.

OTHER POXVIRUS DISEASES

Molluscum contagiosum

A low grade infection in man characterised by reddish, waxy papules on the skin—most often seen in the axilla or on the trunk. It is a fairly common infection in children and is spread by close contact, e.g. at swimming baths; the lesions contain numerous poxvirus particles which can be seen in the electron microscope; the lesions resolve spontaneously in 4 to 6 weeks.

103

Orf or contagious pustular dermatitis

An infection of sheep and goats: occasionally transmitted to hands of animal workers causing chronic granulomatous lesions; diagnosed by characteristic oval particles in electron microscope with criss-cross surface banding.

Paravaccinia or pseudocowpox

The virus appears to be identical with orf virus: it causes lesions on udders of cows and is occasionally transmitted to hands of animal workers.

Monkeypox

This is a disease resembling mild smallpox which is due to a natural pox virus of monkeys; it is seen in Africa among people with frequent contact with monkeys.

Tanapox

This virus is probably also acquired from contact with monkeys and, in humans, produces scanty vesicular lesions on the skin which do not progress to pustules. Epidemics have been reported in East Africa.

Virology

1. Pox viruses include the human viruses smallpox (variola) and molluscum contagiosum, vaccinia (origin uncertain—probably a recombinant virus) together with cowpox and other animal pox viruses.
2. DNA viruses—double-stranded DNA
3. Large viruses, approximately 250–300 nm: two morphological types of particle:
   (i) Large, brick-shaped (Fig. 12.1) (vaccinia, molluscum contagiosum)
   (ii) Large, oval with criss-cross surface bonding (orf, paravaccinia)
4. Some grow in tissue cultures, others do not (e.g. molluscum contagiosum)
5. Many produce characteristic pocks or visible lesions on the chorio-allantoic membrane of the chick embryo.

13

Viral hepatitis

Hepatitis is a complication of infection with many different viruses, e.g. cytomegalovirus, EB virus, and yellow fever virus. However, some viruses primarily infect the liver—namely hepatitis A, hepatitis B and the so-called non-A, non-B hepatitis.

Hepatitis A is a childhood enteric infection but hepatitis B is mainly transmitted parenterally e.g. by blood transfusion: non-A, non-B hepatitis is spread both parenterally and by the faecal-oral route.

All three forms of hepatitis have similar signs and symptoms.

Clinical features

The main symptom is *jaundice* with dark bile-containing urine and pale stools—classical features of obstructive jaundice; liver function tests are abnormal with raised levels of serum aspartate amino transaminase (AST) and serum alanine amino transaminase (ALT); there is low grade fever with nausea—which may be severe—and vomiting. Patients often feel tired and depressed for weeks or even months after the acute attack.

Anicteric hepatitis: is common with all three forms of hepatitis: there is anorexia, malaise and sometimes fever but no jaundice. However, liver function tests are abnormal although liver damage is insufficient to cause frank jaundice.

Symptomless infection: also very common.

Arthralgia and rash: are seen in the prodromal stage of hepatitis B; thought to be serum-sickness-like symptoms (due to immune complexes formed between hepatitis virus and antibody)—although there is usually little antibody at this stage of illness.

Fulminant hepatic failure is a rare but serious complication of hepatitis. In this, centrilobular confluent necrosis leads to massive hepatic necrosis, the patients develop progressive liver failure and the mortality rate is high. A particular problem in pregnancy with non-A, non-B hepatitis.

Viraemia: virus is present in the blood during the acute phase; persistent viraemia is common in hepatitis B but not in hepatitis A in which virus is usually cleared rapidly from the blood after the acute illness.

Virus in faeces: the stools are infectious in hepatitis A; virus is not present in faeces in hepatitis B.

Hepatitis A and B have been extensively studied: the main differences between them are listed in Table 13.1.

Table 13.1 Main differences between hepatitis A and hepatitis B

	Hepatitis A	Hepatitis B
Incubation period	2 to 6 weeks	2 to 5 months
Transmission	faecal-oral	parenteral: close personal contact
Age	mainly schoolchildren	mainly young adult males
Seasonal incidence	autumn and winter	none
Onset	acute	insidious
Clinically	milder	generally more severe
Hepatitis B antigen(s) in blood	no	yes
Persistent infection	no	yes
Mortality rate	0.1–0.2%	low but variable and generally higher than in hepatitis A

HEPATITIS A

Epidemiology

World-wide in distribution: endemic in most countries, more common in rural than urban communities. Epidemics appear from time to time, some of which are associated with sewage contamination of food or water.

Age incidence: mainly affects children aged 5 to 15 years but epidemics are seen in military recruit populations and children's institutions; food-borne outbreaks may involve adults predominantly.

Alimentary infection: the site of entry and of primary multiplication of the virus is the alimentary tract;

Virus is excreted in the faeces for about 2 weeks before the onset of jaundice but for only a few days after the development of symptoms.

Hepatitis is due to spread of virus to the liver (where it replicates in the hepatocytes) in what is primarily an enteric infection.

Antibody to hepatitis A virus appears at the time of onset of jaundice—initially IgM with later but longer persisting IgG.

Spread: there are two main routes of infection:
1. *Case-to-case spread* via the faecal-oral route, the most common route of spread of the disease; symptomless excretors may be an important—because undetected—source of infection.
2. *Via contaminated food and water*: numerous outbreaks have been described due to contamination of food-stuffs by a food-handler who is excreting virus or to pollution of water by infected sewage. *Raw shellfish* (especially oysters) which have become contaminated by growing in sewage-polluted water have been responsible for several large outbreaks.

Decline: the incidence of hepatitis A in Europe (and especially in Britain) declined sharply in the decade of the 1970s, although the disease has increased again in the 1980s. This seems to have been due to some block in the normal faecal-oral route of transmission in children. The decrease in incidence has not been observed in underdeveloped or tropical countries.

Virology

1. A picornavirus: enterovirus 72.
2. RNA (single-stranded) virus

3. Small spherical particles, 27 nm
4. Relatively heat-resistant i.e. withstands 60°C for 30 minutes
5. Does not grow in tissue culture by ordinary methods: some limited multiplication of laboratory adapted strains has been demonstrated in primate cells: there is no CPE
6. Pathogenic for chimpanzees and other primates e.g. marmosets.

Diagnosis

1. *Serology*: detection of virus-specific IgM by radio-immune assay or ELISA.
2. *Demonstration of virus* in stools by electron microscopy.

Passive immunisation

Inoculation of normal immunoglobulin has a protective effect in people exposed to hepatitis A; there is no immunity for 2 weeks after inoculation but the immunity thereafter lasts for 4 to 6 months: recommended for anyone travelling to tropical or Mediterranean countries where hepatitis A is endemic and common.

HEPATITIS B

Epidemiology

Hepatitis B is still the main cause of post-transfusion hepatitis in Britain—now decreasing in incidence as a result of screening blood donations for hepatitis B antigen. Blood may be highly infectious and one extensive epidemic of infection followed the use of yellow fever vaccine during the Second World War which included human serum as a stabilizing agent. Infection can also be spread by the use of communal or inadequately sterilized syringes and needles.

Drug addicts: are at particular risk from hepatitis B; infection is transmitted by sharing of unsterilized syringes used for intravenous administration of drugs: young male drug abusers are the main victims of hepatitis in Britain today and constitute a major health problem at present.

Tattooing and acupuncture: have also been the source of outbreaks of hepatitis B; less obviously, the disease was common amongst *track runners* in Sweden apparently either through communal bathing or by direct inoculation resulting from scratches and minor abrasions caused by running through thickets.

Sexual transmission: patients—especially male homosexuals—attending clinics for sexually-transmitted diseases show a higher incidence of antigen and antibody to the virus than the normal population and the disease itself is more common in male homosexuals—many of whom are also drug abusers—than in other groups in the community.

Non-parenteral spread: although in many cases a source of parenterally-acquired infection can be discovered, some cases appear to be due to non-parenteral transmission—possibly through close personal contact.

Renal dialysis units: hepatitis B has in the past been a particular problem in renal units: infection is introduced by the blood transfusions required by the patients and spreads from them to other patients and staff. The staff involved has been not only doctors and nurses but also biochemistry and haematology M.L.S.O.s who handle samples of infected blood. There have been several outbreaks of infection, some have been mild with no deaths: in others, like that in Edinburgh Royal Infirmary in which there was a 30% case fatality rate, the mortality has been high.

Carriers of hepatitis B virus: in Africa and Asia symptomless carriage is common—up to 15% (and even higher) of some populations: in Britain the incidence of carriage is about 0.1%. There is now good evidence that hepatitis B can cause primary liver cancer and carriers of the virus show a 300-fold increase in the incidence of this tumour (a common form of cancer in tropical countries).

Animal hepatitis B counterparts: a very interesting parallel to human hepatitis B exists in the animal world where some species of ducks, Beechey ground squirrels and woodchucks are natural hosts to similar viruses. A high incidence of primary liver cell cancer is associated with infection in woodchucks and ducks.

Acute hepatitis B in pregnancy: is sometimes followed by infection of the infant; the virus is probably transmitted transplacentally *in utero* towards the end of pregnancy or during delivery; the infected babies become chronic carriers of hepatitis B antigen in their blood and around half of them develop persistent hepatitis. Infection of the newborn infant is less common when the mother is a symptomless carrier of hepatitis B virus or antigen; however, more infants become infected in the months after birth presumably due to close contact with their mothers.

Sequelae of hepatitis B: attacks of acute hepatitis B are followed—in around 3% of cases—by the development of *chronic active hepatitis*; this severe disease is associated with liver dysfunction and a fluctuating course leading in many cases to cirrhosis and progressive liver failure. Not all—in fact probably only a minority of—cases of chronic active hepatitis are due to previous hepatitis B.

Chronic persistent hepatitis is a benign and self-limiting disease which may follow hepatitis B; there are mild inflammatory signs in the liver but symptoms are minor or absent; this disease too is probably associated with previous hepatitis B in a minority of patients.

Virology

Hepatitis B antigen is present in the serum of patients in the acute stage of hepatitis B; in most patients the antigen disappears in convalescence but in about 5% of patients the antigen persists for long periods of time.

Electron microscopy: the antigen consists of three types of particle (Fig. 13.1):
1. Spherical particles 22 nm in diameter.
2. Tubular particles 22 nm in diameter.
3. Larger, spherical particles (known as Dane particles) 42 nm in diameter.

Dane particles are the virions of hepatitis B virus, the smaller 22 nm particles being aggregates of coat protein; Dane particles contain circular double-stranded DNA (but this has quite a large single-stranded region) and have a virion-associated DNA-dependent DNA polymerase.

Antigenic structure: Dane particles have the following antigens:
HBsAg: the surface antigen found also on the 22 nm particles.
HBcAg: the antigen of the inner core of the Dane particle.

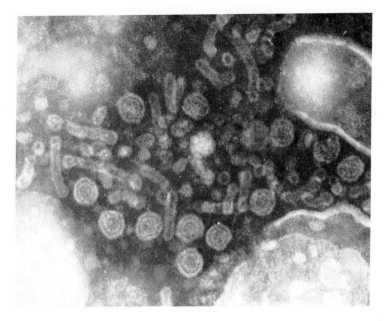

Fig. 13.1 Electron micrographs of hepatitis B virus showing large 42 nm Dane particles, smaller 22 nm spherical and tubular particles. × 220 000 (Photograph by Dr E.A.C. Follett.)

HBeAg: also associated with the core of the Dane particle and correlated with infectivity (see below).

Antigenic subtypes: the 4 subtypes of hepatitis B antigen are based on HBsAg:

adw

adr

ayw

ayr

All share the group-specific determinant *a* in addition to the allelic *d* and *y* (never found together) and—although less often tested—allelic *w* and *r* (which are also mutually exclusive).

Subtype distribution: the predominant subtype of hepatitis B antigen in various situations is as follows:

Symptomless blood donors	*ad*
Acute hepatitis	*ad* and *ay*

Renal units   *ay*
Drug abusers   *ay*

e antigen: this antigen is usually present—although briefly—in patients' blood in the acute phase of hepatitis B; its presence in the blood of cases or carriers correlates with infectivity of the blood. The continuing presence of e antigen also correlates with chronic liver disease and it is found in the blood of a high proportion of patients with chronic active hepatitis following hepatitis B. Conversely: anti-e antibody is usually present in healthy carriers and the infectivity of blood containing it is low.

Antibody to hepatitis B core antigen (HBcAb) appears early in infection whereas *antibody to hepatitis B surface antigen* (HBsAb) appears later during convalescence: antibody to hepatitis B surface antigen is present in about 3 to 9% of the normal population. The incidence is higher in certain groups, e.g. in people with a past history of hepatitis B and hospital staff members.

Diagnosis

Serology

Detection of hepatitis B surface antigen (HBsAg)—tests:
1. *Radio-immune assay*—the most sensitive test.
2. ELISA: almost as sensitive as radio-immune assay.
3. *Reversed passive haemagglutination*: turkey erythrocytes are coated with hepatitis B antibody prepared in horses; the patient's serum is then tested for haemagglutination with these cells.
4. *Counter immunoelectroosmophoresis* was formerly widely used for detection of hepatitis B antigen. It has been superceded by more sensitive methods of detection.

Additional useful tests:
1. Detection of HBcAb (IgM) by ELISA
2. Detection of e antigen (HBeAg) by radio-immune assay or ELISA.

Tests of immunity (or previous infection)
1. Detection of hepatitis B antibody by radio-immune assay or ELISA.

Passive immunization: injection of hepatitis B-specific immunoglobulin gives partial but significant protection against the disease: it should be used in people exposed in a single episode involving a high risk of infection e.g. accidental inoculation of blood suspected or known to contain hepatitis Bs antigen.

Delta agent: is a defective RNA virus found only in the presence of hepatitis B. Hepatitis B virus acts as a helper in its replication and delta agent contains hepatitis B surface antigen as the outer coat of its particle. Found mainly in drug abusers and multiply-transfused patients, its role in disease is uncertain.

Vaccine

Now available for those at special risk (e.g. virology laboratory staff, patients and staff in institutions for the mentally subnormal, renal units, babies born to carrier mothers).

Contains: inactivated HbsAg purified from the blood of carriers.

Administered: subcutaneously in three doses at intervals of one and then six months.
Protection: apparently good
Safety: good
Note: a vaccine containing genetically-engineered HbsAg is under trial.

Non-A, non B-hepatitis

When it became possible to diagnose both hepatitis A and B in the laboratory, it became clear that there was a third form of hepatitis of which the causal virus was unrelated to either hepatitis A or hepatitis B viruses. Known as non-A, non-B the disease comprises at least three forms of viral hepatitis:

1. Transmitted by blood transfusion or by injection of blood products
2. Sporadic or endemic hepatitis
3. Epidemic water-borne hepatitis

The causal agents appear to be unrelated to each other and to hepatitis A or B.

Widespread epidemics of water-borne non-A, non-B hepatitis have been reported in India. Infection is by the faecal-oral route due to sewage contamination of the water supply. The disease is generally mild except in pregnant women in whom there is a high mortality due to the frequent development of fulminant hepatitis.

14

Antiviral therapy

Virus infections cannot be treated specifically—with a few exceptions—in the same way as antibiotics have been used so successfully for bacterial diseases. The few antiviral drugs that have been developed are mainly for herpesvirus infections.

Note: Viruses are resistant to all antibacterial antibiotics.

Below are some of the principle antiviral drugs;

PURINE AND PYRIMIDINE NUCLEOSIDES

1. Acyclovir—acycloguanosine
2. Idoxuridine—5-iodo-2-deoxyuridine
3. Cytarabine—cytosine arabinoside
4. Vidarabine—adenine arabinoside

ACYCLOVIR

Acyclovir is somewhat of a break-through in antiviral therapy since it is non-toxic to cells but extremely inhibitory to virus replication. It has virtually replaced the other nucleosides for herpes infections.

Viruses inhibited: herpes simplex, varicella-zoster: not active against cytomegalovirus.

Action: inhibition of virus DNA synthesis: acyclovir is phosphorylated by herpes-specific thymidine kinase to monophosphate and it is this form which acts to inhibit virus DNA polymerase: since it is inactive in uninfected cells it shows minimal toxicity.

Administration: intravenous, oral, topical

Side effects: transient depression of renal function in an occasional patient.

Indications for use (see also chapter 10)

Treatment

1. Herpes simplex encephalitis, severe cold sores in the immuno-compromised, genital herpes
2. Dendritic ulcer and cold sores (topically)
3. Zoster—especially severe zoster in the immuno-compromised.

Prophylaxis

1. Herpes simplex (and zoster) reactivation in the immunocom-promised (e.g. renal, bone marrow, heart transplant recipients).

The introduction of acyclovir has diminished the indications for the other nucleosides. However they are still in use for some infections.

IDOXURIDINE

Not used now for systemic therapy because of toxicity. Still used for treatment of herpes simplex dendritic ulcer by topical application and possibly also to zoster lesions.

VIDARABINE

Of proven efficacy in herpes encephalitis (although there was a high incidence of sequelae in survivors) but now replaced by acyclovir as therapy for that disease. Used topically for herpes simplex dendritic ulcers and systemically for zoster in the immuno-compromised.

INTERFERON

Interferon is still a promising antiviral agent: relatively non-toxic (but it has some pyrogen-like side-effects), active against all viruses, it may yet prove to be an effective and practicable way of treating and preventing virus infections: quantities of human interferon are still limited, although genetically-engineered preparations may soon become available.

Interferon is not a single substance but a family of cellular molecules with regulatory functions which not only inhibit virus replication, but have multiple effects on cell metabolism as well.

There are three main types of human interferon (HuIFN):
1. IFN—α: produced by human leucocytes: formerly known as Le (leucocyte) type I interferon
2. IFN—β: produced by human fibroblasts: formerly known as F (fibroblast) type I interferon
3. IFN—γ: produced by human lymphocytes in response to antigenic or mitogenic stimulation: formerly known as type II (immune) interferon.

Properties

Cellular protein(s): interferon is a family of cell regulatory molecules released from cells in response to virus infection (and probably to other stimuli also); when interferon is taken up by uninfected cells these become resistant to virus infection; it is produced by cells in tissue culture as well as in intact animals.

Induction: interferon is produced in response to inactivated as well as live viruses; RNA viruses are better inducers than DNA viruses. Synthetic polyribonucleotides are powerful inducers: polyribo-inosinic-polyribocytidylic acid (poly rI: poly rC) is a particularly good inducer.

Species-specific: interferon is active only in cells of the same animal species in which it was formed.

Virus susceptibility: all viruses are inhibited by interferon but RNA viruses are generally more susceptible than DNA viruses.

Mode of action: interferon binds to the cell plasma membrane; in cells treated with interferon, viral nucleic acid and protein synthesis are inhibited; adsorption, penetration and uncoating take place normally.

Interferon has two main actions:
1. *Degradation of mRNA* by an endonuclease which is activated by the oligonucleotide 2, 5 A. The oligonucleotide is itself synthesized by the stimulation of a synthetase activated by the combined effect of interferon and double-stranded RNA.

2. *Inhibition of protein synthesis.* Interferon and double-stranded RNA also activate a protein kinase which in turn phosphorylates and so inactivates the initiation factor in protein synthesis, eIF-2.

Effect on human virus infections: interferon administered intranasally prevents experimentally-induced rhinovirus infection; it also prevents vaccinia infection if injected intradermally at the site of inoculation. In clinical trials it appears to have an effect—but not a dramatic one—in herpes keratitis, zoster, cytomegalovirus infection, and chronic active hepatitis due to hepatitis B virus.

Effect in cancer: clinical trials with interferon have shown a significant effect in several human tumours such as osteogenic sarcoma, myeloma, lymphoma and breast cancer. Most available supplies of interferon are therefore at present being used for trials in cancer patients.

AMANTADINE (1-adamantine hydrochloride)

Amantadine can prevent influenza A—both naturally-occurring and experimentally-induced; it acts by blocking the penetration of influenza A virus into cells but has no effect on influenza B virus. It is administered orally; side-effects may follow its use—these involve the central nervous system and particularly affect elderly patients; amantadine has never become widely used.

15

Slow virus diseases

Slow virus diseases are classically defined as diseases with a long incubation period, slow development of symptoms and a protracted, sometimes fatal course. Some are chronic infections with conventional viruses but others are due to unconventional agents which may be viruses but are certainly quite unlike most human pathogenic viruses. Examples of slow virus diseases in man due to conventional viruses are listed in Table 15.1. There are many examples in animals due to a variety of different viruses.

Table 15.1 Slow virus diseases due to conventional viruses

Virus	Disease
Measles	Subacute sclerosing panencephalitis
Rubella	Subacute sclerosing panencephalitis (follows congenital infection)
J C (human polyoma virus)	Progressive multifocal leucoencephalopathy.
Hepatitis B	Hepatitis B, chronic active and chronic persistent hepatitis.

Most of the diseases in Table 15.1. have been described in earlier chapters on the appropriate viruses. Progressive multifocal leucoencephalopathy is described below:

PROGRESSIVE MULTIFOCAL LEUCOENCEPHALOPATHY

This rare disease is now regarded as a slow virus disease due to a conventional virus—in this instance the papovavirus known as JC or human polyoma virus: it is opportunistic in that it is only seen in patients whose health is compromised by pre-existing disease such as leukaemia, reticulosis or immuno-suppressive therapy.

Clinical features

Varied neurological signs: such as hemiparesis, dementia, dysphasia, incoordination, impaired vision and hemianaesthesia.

Duration: usually fatal in 3 to 4 months.

Pathology: multiple foci of demyelination in cerebral haemispheres and cerebellum: brain stem and basal ganglia may also be affected.

Histology: oligodendrocytes with swollen nuclei and intranuclear inclusions are characteristic features.

Epidemiology

Infection with the virus is widespread in the community and a considerable proportion of people have antibody to it; it does not cause disease in normal people and progressive multifocal leucoencephalopathy is a rare complication due to reactivation of latent virus in an immunocompromised host.

Virology

JC virus has the following properties:
1. Typical papovirus morphology
2. Contains circular, double-stranded DNA
3. Grows in human fetal glial tissue cultures; virus growth is recognised by electron microscopy
4. Haemagglutinates human and guinea pig erythrocytes at 4°C.

Note: the other human polyoma virus—*BK virus*—is also an opportunistic pathogen. It has been isolated from immunodeficient patients, presumably due to reactivation of latent virus. Like JC virus, BK antibody is present in a high proportion of human populations so that symptomless infection seems to be widespread.

Oncogenicity: both JC and BK viruses transform cells in tissue culture.

SLOW VIRUS DISEASES DUE TO UNCONVENTIONAL AGENTS

There are three slow virus diseases, all of which involve the CNS, and which are due to unconventional agents. These are clearly not typical viruses—prions or infectious proteins have been suggested: they have never been seen in the electron microscope.

Infections with the agents show the following features:

1. Long incubation period
2. Protracted, severe, progressive course: virtually always fatal
3. Pathology: degeneration of the CNS with status spongiosus
4. Lesions show no inflammatory reaction
5. No antibody or other immune response.

Three slow virus diseases of this type are listed in Table 15.2.

Table 15.2 Slow virus diseases due to unconventional agents.

Virus	Host species	Pathological features	Disease syndrome
Kuru	Man	Subacute cerebellar degeneration; status spongiosus	Postural instability; ataxia, tremor
Creutzfeldt-Jakob disease	Man	Subacute degeneration of brain and spinal cord with status spongiosus of cortex	Presenile dementia; ataxia, spasticity, involuntary movements
Scrapie	Sheep	Subacute cerebellar degeneration	Ataxia, tremor, constant rubbing; susceptibility to infection is genetically determined

SCRAPIE

Scrapie is a neurological disease of sheep common in Britain 200 years ago and now present in sheep in many other countries also. Because of strong evidence that it is due to an infectious agent about the size of a small virus, it has been the subject of a great deal of research.

Clinical features

Natural scrapie affects both sheep and goats; the following are features of natural scrapie in sheep:

Long incubation period: from 2 to 5 years.

Signs and symptoms: affected sheep suffer from excitability, incoordination, ataxia, tremor and continous scratching or rubbing due to sensory neurological disturbance; the symptoms progress to paralysis and death.

Pathology: cerebellar neuronal degeneration with astrocytic proliferation; status spongiosus.

Heredity: a major gene controls whether or not sheep develop disease after experimental inoculation; the operation of the gene is complex and depends partly on the strain of agent used for inoculation.

Route of infection: the disease is transmitted by contact in flocks of sheep and also vertically from ewes to lambs.

Scrapie agent

Scrapie can be transmitted by intracerebral or subcutaneous inoculation using the brains of infected sheep. The incubation period varies from 3 to 24 months depending on the strain of agent; the disease can also be transmitted to and passaged in mice with a shorter incubation period of 4 to 8 weeks; experimental infection in mice forms the basic technique of assaying the agent.

Properties of the scrapie agent

1. Small size—20 to 30 nm
2. Resistant to ultraviolet-irradiation, formaldehyde and heat (e.g. resists 80° for 60 minutes)
3. Does not stimulate antibody production in experimental animals.

   No nucleic acid has been demonstrated in the scrapie agent nor has it been seen by electron microscopy; the remarkable resistance to ultraviolet-irradiation suggests that, if nucleic acid is present, it must be in small amounts.

TRANSMISSABLE MINK ENCEPHALOPATHY

A disease due to scrapie agent: mink bred in mink farms have become infected when fed on the heads of scrapie-infected sheep.

KURU

Kuru is a fatal human disease found only among the Foré-speaking people in New Guinea. It seems to have appeared about 60 years ago. The incidence increased up until the late 1950s when kuru was responsible for about half the deaths in the Foré-speaking people. The incidence of kuru declined rapidly in the early 1960s.

Clinical features

1. *Kuru* is a native word meaning 'trembling with cold and fever'.
2. *The first or ambulant stage* of the disease starts with unsteadiness in walking, postural instability, ataxia and tremor; facial expressions are poorly controlled and speech becomes slurred and tremulous.
3. *The second or sedentary stage* is reached when the patient cannot walk without support, but can still sit upright unaided.
4. *In the tertiary stage the patient cannot sit upright* without clutching a stick for support; even a gentle push makes the patient lurch violently; the patient becomes progressively more paralysed and emaciated.
5. *Duration* of the disease averages one year but ranges from three months to two years.
6. *Death* is due to bulbar depression or intercurrent infection.
7. *Pathology*: neuronal degeneration in cerebellum with astrocytic hyperplasia, gliosus and status spongiosus; demyelination is minimal or absent.
8. *Sex incidence*: kuru is uncommon in adult males; most patients are women or children of both sexes.
9. *Cannibalism of dead relatives* is thought to have been responsible for the spread of kuru among the Foré people. Men do not usually take part in these cannibalistic feasts. The women and children eat the viscera and brains of relatives including those who have died of kuru. This unusual cultural habit seems to have been responsible for the spread of infection. Spread may have been through contact of infected tissues with abrasions on skin rather than, or as well as, ingestion. The tissues are inadequately cooked so the causal agent would not be inactivated by cooking.
10. *Cannibalism stopped around 1957* and kuru has now declined sharply in incidence: this supports the theory that the disease has been spread by cannibalism; on the assumption that kuru is apread in this way, the *incubation period* appears to be from 4 to 20 years.

Causal agent

Transmission experiments: intracerebral inoculation of brain tissue from kuru victims into chimpanzees and other monkeys causes the animals to develop the symptoms of kuru after an incubation period of two years. After passage, the incubation period is shortened to about one year.

The reproduction of the disease in experimental animals is strong evidence that kuru is due to an infectious agent. However, attempts to cultivate the causal agent from both human and chimpanzee tissues in tissue cultures have been unsuccessful.

Experimental studies in chimpanzees have shown that the agent has the following properties:

1. *Passes filters* of 100 nm pore diameter—indicating that it is in the size range of viruses
2. *Present in infected brain tissue* to a titre of 10^6 infectious units per ml
3. *Present in spleen, liver and kidney* of infected animals although the organs appear normal
4. *Can be transmitted peripherally* (i.e. by combined intravenous, subcutaneous, intramuscular and intraperitoneal routes) as well as intracerebrally
5. *No antibody* to the agent has been detected in either humans or chimpanzees with kuru.

CREUTZFELDT-JAKOB DISEASE

A rare progressive neurological disease characterized by a combination of presenile dementia with symptoms due to lesions in the spinal cord.

Clinical features

1. *Prodromal stage*: the disease starts with tiredness, apathy and vague neurological symptoms
2. *Second stage*: the patient develops ataxia, dysarthria and progressive spasticity of the limbs, this is associated with dementia and often involuntary movements such as myoclonic jerks or choreoathetoid movements
3. *The disease progresses steadily* until death—usually from about six months to two years after the onset of symptoms
4. *Pathology*: diffuse atrophy with status spongiosus in the cerebral

cortex; atrophy also in basal ganglia, cerebellum, substantia nigra and anterior horn cells.

Causal agent

Transmission experiments: the disease is reproduced in chimpanzees and other monkeys after intracerebral inoculation of brain tissue from cases of the disease; the incubation period is from 11 to 14 months; the disease can also be transmitted peripherally (by combined intravenous, intraperitoneal and intramuscular routes).

Human infection: the natural route of infection is unknown but Creutzfeldt-Jakob disease has been accidentally transmitted via a corneal graft to the recipient. Transmission has also been reported by electrodes used for electro-encephalography from a patient with the disease to other patients in whom the electrodes were subsequently implanted. Recently, transmission of the disease has been reported in patients injected with growth hormone derived from human pituitary gland.

Note: slow virus diseases due to unconventional agents are attracting considerable interest because of the possibility that certain human neurological diseases of unknown cause (e.g. multiple sclerosis, amyotrophic lateral sclerosis, Altzheimer's disease) might be due to similar agents.

16

Tumour viruses

Knowledge of the molecular basis of cancer is advancing rapidly at present and tumour viruses are the tools that have made this possible.

A variety of different viruses cause tumours in animals. Because their genetics and replicative processes are relatively well understood, events at the molecular level of carcinogenesis are now being discovered. Knowledge of this is still incomplete but it seems likely that the next few years will bring about a greater understanding of the causes of human cancer—and hopefully—prevention or cure.

Tumour viruses include:
1. RNA viruses (retroviruses)
2. DNA viruses of various different families.

The oncogenicity of a virus can be shown in two ways:
1. Inoculation of the virus into experimental animals produces tumours.
2. The virus transforms normal cells in tissue culture into cells with characteristics of malignant or cancer cells.

Transformation of cells in tissue culture

Transformation of cells in tissue culture is believed to be analogous to the induction by viruses of cancer in intact animals. Transformed cells have virus-specific DNA (which may represent the whole or only a fragment of the virus genome) integrated into the cell chromosome.

Transformed cells show the following altered properties from normal cells:
1. *Morphological change*
2. *Loss of contact inhibition*: normal cells stop dividing when they form a monolayer and come in contact with neighbouring cells;

transformed cells grow unrestrainedly and pile up into dense layers

3. *Growth in agar*: normal cells cannot divide when suspended in semi-solid agar
4. *Increased agglutinability* with the plant lectin concanavalin A
5. *New antigens* which may or may not be virus-specified
6. *Transplantability*: transformed cells show enhanced ability to produce tumours on inoculation into experimental animals.

RETROVIRUSES

Many retroviruses cause natural cancer in the host animal. They also produce tumours—which are mainly leukaemia or sarcomas—or inoculation into experimental animals. Although sarcoma viruses transform cells most of the leukaemia viruses do not.

Morphology

Retroviruses have similar but also slightly different types of particle:

1. C-type particles: Most retroviruses have spherical enveloped particles surrounded by spikes or knobs and containing a central core composed of RNA and protein (Fig. 16.1).
2. B-type particles: Mouse mammary tumour virus (also a retrovirus) has particles similar to C-type particles but with an eccentric core or nucleoid.
3. D-type particles: have typical retrovirus morphology but with a central cylindrical core, and are typified by Mason-Pfizer Monkey virus and the newly discovered AIDS-related human retrovirus HTLV III.

Note All retrovirus particles contain the enzyme reverse transcriptase (see Chapter 2).

Genome structure

The retrovirus genome contains four genes:

1. The *gag* gene—codes for the core protein antigens of the virus particle. These are cleaved from a larger precursor protein
2. The *pol* gene—codes for the protein that is the reverse transcriptase

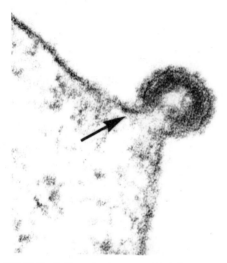

Fig. 16.1 Feline leukaemia virus—a typical C-type retrovirus particle budding through the plasma membrane on its release from the cell. The continuity between the cell surface membrane and the virion is indicated by the arrow and the spikes on the surface of the outer virion membrane are clearly seen. ×190 000 (Photograph by Dr. Helen Laird).

3. The *env* gene—codes for the glycoprotein envelope proteins of the virion
4. The *onc* gene—responsible for transformation.

Transformation

The *onc* gene of retroviruses codes for a protein which is responsible for transformation. In the avian retrovirus, Rous sarcoma virus, this protein is an enzyme which phosphorylates tyrosine residues and probably affects cell regulation and so produces malignant transformation of cells (see also Chapter 2).

Oncogenes

Oncogenes are genes whose expression can be associated with tumour production. It is now clear that these are present as a result of vertical inheritance in many normal cells. Retroviruses cause cancer when their genome acquires cellular oncogenes by recombination. This probably happens when RNA tumour viruses integrate in the form of provirus DNA into cellular chromosomes. Numerous oncogenes have been described in animal retroviruses. In these cases their designation is preceded by the letter 'v' e.g. v-*myc* or v-*ras*: their cellular counterparts are known as c-*myc* or c-*ras*. Activated cellular oncogenes may differ by only a single base mutation from their normal progenitor gene. Oncogenes do not always give rise to carcinogenesis. They need to be activated and different mechanisms can be responsible for this:

1. a virus promoter such as that contained in the long terminal repeat region of the retrovirus genome
2. a cellular promoter—possibly by translocation to a site on a chromosome with high activity
3. a co-factor such as a chemical carcinogen
4. interaction with other oncogenes.

It seems likely that oncogenes normally function as regulatory mechanisms in cells: their activation to produce tumours is probably the result of a loss of control of normal gene function leading to disturbance of the usual regulatory activity.

Epidemiology

Most animal species (including man) in which a detailed search has been made are natural hosts for retroviruses that are characteristic of the species.

Transmission

Transmission from animal to animal takes place in three ways:

1. *Horizontal*: in which the virus spreads by direct contact, or possibly inhalation, between infected and susceptible animals. This is an important route in naturally-occurring infection in outbred animals not reared in a laboratory, such as cats.
2. *Congenital*: vertical transmission in which the virus spreads from mother to offspring either by infection *in utero* or via the mother's milk.
3. *Genetic*: also vertical transmission but in this case the virus is inherited in the form of a provirus or viral DNA transcript inte-

grated into the chromosomes of the germ cells of the parent animal. The viruses produced from proviruses are known as *endogenous* viruses and are typical retroviruses: however, although some are tumour-producing on inoculation into experimental animals, many are not. Endogenous retroviruses are usually present in a repressed state but can be induced by various agents so that their genes are derepressed with consequent production of the virus in the animal.

Endogenous retroviruses are present in normal cells of chickens, mice, cats and some primates.

TUMOURS PRODUCED BY RETROVIRUSES

Most retroviruses which cause tumours in animals can be divided into:
1. Sarcoma viruses
2. Leukaemia viruses

Sarcoma viruses

Sarcoma viruses readily transform cells in tissue culture and produce solid tumours—fibrosarcomas—on inoculation into animals of the host species. Most are defective so that, in order to replicate, they require the presence of a helper virus (usually a leukaemia virus of the same animal species) to supply the product of the defective gene. The defective viruses have deletions in one or more of the three structural genes, often because host genes with oncogenic potential have been substituted in their place. The deletion often involves the *env* gene and as a result sarcoma viruses have the same type-specific neutralizing antigen in their envelope as the helper leukaemia virus.

Leukaemia viruses

Leukaemia viruses produce leukaemia on inoculation into animals. Many do not transform cells in tissue culture although some do so. Leukaemia viruses are not defective and generally replicate in tissue culture. They do not produce CPE and cell growth and division are not affected.

Table 16.1 lists the principle retroviruses, their host animal species and the tumours produced.

Table 16.1 Retroviruses

Host Animal	Virus	Tumour
Chickens	Rous sarcoma virus Avian leukosis viruses	Sarcoma in chickens Fowl leukaemia
Mice	Murine sarcoma virus Murine leukaemia viruses Mouse mammary tumour virus	Sarcoma in mice Mouse leukaemia Breast cancer in mice
Cats	Feline sarcoma virus Feline leukaemia virus	Sarcoma in cats Cat leukaemia
Primates	Simian sarcoma virus Gibbon ape leukaemia virus	Sarcoma in marmosets Leukaemia in gibbon apes
Man	HTLV	T-cell leukaemia

HUMAN RETROVIRUSES

The discovery of these viruses is a major breakthrough in human cancer research and clinical virology. Three have been described, all of which are tropic (i.e. preferentially infect) human T-lymphocytes and are therefore known as human T-cell lymphotropic viruses (HTLV).

HTLV-I   causes T-cell lymphoma in Japan, the Caribbean (and perhaps elsewhere as well)

HTLV-II   isolated from a case of hairy-cell leukaemia

HTLV-III causes acquired immune-deficiency syndrome (AIDS)

Virology

1. Typical retrovirus particles. HTLV-I and II have C-type particles, HTLV-III has D-type particles with a cylindrical rather than circular core.
2. RNA viruses with typical retrovirus genome structure.
3. Grow in T4 helper lymphocytes: HTLV-I and II cause proliferation, HTLV-III is cytopathic.
4. Culture: can be cultivated in continuous cell lines of human lymphocytes growing as suspension cultures (i.e. the cells do not adhere to form monolayers on glass or plastic surfaces).

HTLV-I and II

Both viruses have been isolated from lymphoid malignancies. HTLV-I, the commoner of the two, causes T-cell lymphomas which are frequent tumours in Southern Japan and the Caribbean. In these areas, the normal population have a high incidence of virus antibody. Recent work suggests that T-cell lymphomas elsewhere, including Britain, may also be associated with infection with HTLV-I. The ecology of HTLV-II is unknown.

HTLV-III

The cause of AIDS, a new disease of severe immune deficiency and now rapidly increasing in incidence in the USA and Western Europe. The virus probably originated in central Africa.

Clinical

1. Most infections are probably symptomless.
2. The earliest symptoms, around a month after infection, are self-limiting and similar to those of infectious mononucleosis.
3. After a variable but often prolonged incubation period (6 months to 6 years), persistent generalised lymphadenopathy (PGL) may develop. In many, perhaps most patients, PGL resolves without further symptoms.
4. In a few patients, the infection progresses to the AIDS-related complex (ARC) in which the patient feels ill with tiredness, weight loss, anaemia, chronic diarrhoea: some opportunistic infections such as herpes simplex or candida appear. ARC generally progresses to the full-blown AIDS.
5. AIDS
   A disease characterized by:
   i. Opportunistic infections
   ii. Kaposi's sarcoma
   iii. Inversion of normal T4:T8 ratios of lymphocyte subsets due to depletion of T4 helper lymphocytes.

i. Opportunistic infections

Most common: Pneumocystis carinii pneumonia.
Others described include: herpes simplex, candida, cytomegalovirus, zoster, toxoplasmosis, cryptosporidiosis, infection with *Mycobacterium* species (typical and atypical).

ii. Kaposi's sarcoma

A rare tumour in Western Europe and USA, but seen in about a quarter of AIDS cases and in an unusually aggressive form.

Cerebral lymphoma

Another rare tumour which should arouse suspicion of AIDS.

Note: AIDS patients commonly suffer from encephalopathy due to infection of the CNS by HTLV-III.

Source of infection

Semen, blood, (virus is present in saliva but this does not seem to be infectious). Virus can be isolated from body secretions and blood of patients who are symptomless but who have HTLV-III antibody as well as those suffering from AIDS.

Routes of infection:

Rectal intercourse, transfusion or inoculation of blood products.

At risk

Homosexual men, haemophiliacs, bisexual men and their partners, Haitians, drug abusers.

Diagnosis

Serological

Detection of HTLV-III antibody by ELISA or immunofluorescence

Blood

Detection of lymphopenia with T4 lymphocyte depletion.

DNA TUMOUR VIRUSES

Unlike retroviruses, many of the most highly oncogenic do not cause naturally-occurring cancer in the host animal. Nevertheless they efficiently produce tumours on inoculation into laboratory animals and transform cells in tissue culture. They are therefore excellent model systems for the investigation of the molecular basis of viral carcinogenesis.

Replication

In permissive cells (i.e. cells in which they can grow) DNA tumour viruses replicate and cause CPE in much the same way as non-oncogenic viruses; however, they tend to stimulate cellular DNA synthesis instead of switching it off as non-tumour viruses do.

Transformation

DNA tumour viruses transform non-permissive cells in which they cannot replicate; cells transformed by DNA viruses do not shed virus like retrovirus-transformed cells. Although in some cases the whole DNA virus genome is integrated into the host cell chromosome, in most only a small fragment of virus DNA is present.

Animal DNA tumour viruses

Among the most studied are polyoma virus of mice, which produces multiple primary tumours in hamsters, and the simian virus SV_{40}. SV_{40} contaminated many of the early batches of polio vaccine which were grown in monkey kidney cells. As a result thousands of children were accidentally injected with live SV_{40}: happily no increase in cancer among them has been observed. Neither polyoma virus nor SV_{40} cause naturally-occurring cancer in mice or monkeys but Marek's disease virus of chickens is a herpes virus which does cause malignant neurolymphomatosis (or Marek's disease) in the host chickens.

Human oncogenic DNA viruses

Human adenoviruses cause sarcomas on inoculation into hamsters—and transform cells in tissue culture—but are not associated with human cancer. Similarly, the human polyoma viruses, JC and BK, are oncogenic *in vitro* and *in vivo* but have not been linked with naturally-occurring tumours.

Table 16.2 Human DNA viruses with oncogenic potential

Virus	Virus Family	Association with Human Cancer
Hepatitis B	Unclassified	Primary liver cell cancer
Epstein Barr (EBV)	Herpes	Burkitt's lymphoma: nasopharyngeal carcinoma
Herpes simplex type 2	Herpes	? cervical cancer
Human papilloma (HPV)	Papova	? cervical cancer
BK/JC human polyoma	Papova	none: *in vitro* and *in vivo* oncogenicity
Adenoviruses	Adenovirus	none: *in vitro* and *in vivo* oncogenicity

Table 16.2 lists the main human DNA viruses with oncogenic potential:

DNA VIRUSES AND HUMAN CANCER

Hepatitis B and Primary liver cell cancer

This cancer is a common malignancy in Africa and the Far East but is rare in Western populations. Areas of high incidence coincide with those where there is a high level of carriage of hepatitis B virus (see also Chapter 13) and carriers have a greatly increased risk of developing liver cancer.

At the molecular level, liver cancer cells contain integrated hepatitis B DNA in their chromosomes. Further strong evidence of a causal link between virus and tumour has been the discovery that viruses very similar to hepatitis B exist naturally in animals and that, in them too, the virus is associated with liver cancer (see also Chapter 13).

EB virus and Burkitt's lymphoma

A highly malignant tumour which is common in African children. Primarily a tumour of lymphoid tissue but the earliest manifestations are often large tumours of the jaw and, in girls, sometimes of the ovaries; it spreads rapidly with widespread metastases.

There is a striking *geographical distribution*: the tumour is virtually confined to areas in Africa in which disease-carrying insect vectors are found. Outside Africa, e.g. in Western Europe and the USA, reported cases are sporadic and rare.

EB virus is almost certainly the cause of Burkitt's lymphoma; the virus is found in cell cultures established from Burkitt's lymphoma and EB virus DNA is present—although not integrated—in the lymphoblasts of the tumour. Patients with Burkitt's lymphoma uniformly have antibody to the virus but so do a high proportion of normal people in any part of the world. Infection with EB virus *per se* does not, therefore, cause Burkitt's lymphoma.

The geographical distribution may be because the areas where Burkitt's lymphoma is found are also areas in which the population is heavily infected with malaria. The effect of the parasites on the reticulo-endothelial system could cause an abnormal response to infection with EB virus. Instead of producing a benign proliferation of lymphoid tissue (as in infectious mononucleosis) the virus may become frankly oncogenic to produce malignant transformation in lymphoid tissue (as in Burkitt's lymphoma).

Nasopharyngeal carcinoma: is a tumour which shows a striking racial or genetic incidence. For example, it is particularly common among the Southern Chinese. Nasopharyngeal carcinoma also seems to be associated with EB virus and virus DNA is regularly present in the malignant epithelial cells of the tumour.

Viruses and cancer of the cervix

The epidemiology of this cancer shows a strong association with sexual activity and multiple sexual partners—factors which suggest a possible infectious aetiology. The two candidate viruses are type 2 herpes simplex and human papilloma virus (HPV) but the evidence incriminating them is far from solid. Women with cervical cancer have a higher incidence of antibodies to type 2 herpes simplex virus than comparable groups of matched control women. Type 2 herpes simplex virus does not produce tumours when inoculated into experimental rodents but it transforms rodent embryo cells in tissue culture and the transformed cells cause tumours on inoculation into experimental animals.

Histologically, small flat warts are surprisingly common in the cervix and can be found in about a third of all women examined. The types of wart virus most often found are HPV types 6, 11, 16 and 18. Molecular hybridization with HPV DNA has demonstrated the presence of HPV DNA in cervical cancer cells. HPV types 16 and 18 are the types most strongly associated with cervical carcinoma: types 6 and 11 seem to have a lower risk of progression to malignancy.

WARTS

Warts are ubiquitous in most species of animal. Warts are skin tumours due to proliferation of epithelial cells. Most regress spontaneously but they are notoriously difficult to treat. Certain types of wart occasionally become cancerous but the vast majority are entirely benign.

Papillomaviruses: Warts are due to the large family of papillomaviruses which are specific for the various animal species which are their natural host.

Shope papilloma virus is of unusual interest: it is the cause of papillomas in wild rabbits and is normally spread by insect vectors; papillomas are produced when the virus is inoculated into wild rabbits and in these tumours cancerous change is relatively rare. In domestic rabbits, Shope papilloma virus produces a higher incidence of papillomas and cancerous changes are observed far more often. Virus cannot be cultured from the tumours that have undergone cancerous change.

HUMAN WARTS

Clinical features

Divided into four categories depending on their clinical appearance and site:

1. *Skin*: especially of the hands and feet (plantar warts): plantar warts sometimes become epidemic in children as a result of cross-infection acquired in swimming baths. Skin warts never undergo malignant change.
2. *Genital* (*condylomata acuminata*): usually transmitted by sexual intercourse, genital warts sometimes become very large. Rarely, they undergo cancerous change
3. *Oral*: warts on the buccal mucosa are rare in Britain but not uncommon in American Indians and Eskimos
4. *Laryngeal papillomas* are also rare in Britain but are common in other areas, e.g. Southern USA. Most often seen in children and sometimes in infants due to infection acquired at birth from genital warts in the mother. Laryngeal papillomas do not become malignant but they tend to recur causing progressive damage to the vocal cords.

Virology

1. Papovaviruses, contain double-stranded circular DNA
2. Typical papovavirus morphology on electron microscopy (Fig. 16.2) but larger (50 nm) than polyoma or SV_{40} viruses (40 nm)
3. Cannot be cultured *in vitro* or *in vivo* (i.e. in experimental laboratory animals)
4. Different types of human wart virus can be distinguished by biochemical techniques (restriction enzyme DNA analysis, DNA hybridization). Different clinical kinds of wart are associated with particular types of virus.

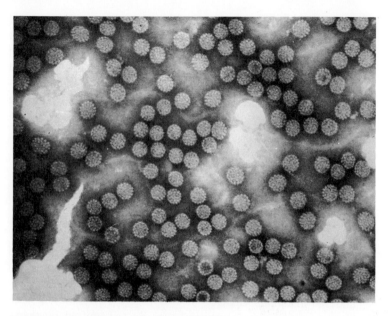

Fig. 16.2 HPV virus. The virus particles have cubic symmetry.
× 90 000 (Photograph by Dr E. A. C. Follett)

17

Chlamydial diseases

Chlamydia are widespread in human and animal populations. They are not viruses although, by tradition, they are usually handled in virus laboratories. They are really bacteria but differ from bacteria in being unable to grow on inanimate media. They are sensitive to tetracycline and erythromycin.

There are two species of *Chlamydia*:
1. *Chlamydia trachomatis*
2. *Chlamydia psittaci*

Below, in Table 17.1, are details of their serotypes and associated diseases.

Table 17.1 Chlamydia

Species	Hosts	Main diseases	Serotypes
Chlamydia trachomatis	Man	Oculogenital	D, E, F, G, H, I, J, K.
		Trachoma Lymphogranuloma venereum	A, B, Ba, C. 1, 2, 3.
Chlamydia psittaci	Various animals (including birds)	Psittacosis	—

Bacteriology of chlamydia

1. Contain both DNA and RNA
2. Larger than most viruses, 250–500 nm: visible by light microscopy
3. Replicate only within living cells: the growth cycle is complex and includes a stage of binary fusion
4. Grow in tissue culture: best cultivated in McCoy or HeLa 229 cells treated with cycloheximide or idoxuridine to stop cell division: chlamydial growth is recognised by the development of intracytoplasmic inclusions detected by Giemsa staining

139

5. Grow in yolk sac of chick embryos
6. Sensitive to tetracycline, erythromycin, sulphonamides.

CHLAMYDIA TRACHOMATIS

Chlam. trachomatis is widespread as a genital infection in human populations and is generally transmitted by sexual intercourse. Infection in women is usually symptomless but, in men, it is responsible for about half the cases of non-specific genital infection. It also causes eye disease, pneumonia, and another sexually transmitted disease—lymphogranuloma venereum.

1. Non-specific genital infection

Also known as non-specific urethritis and by far the commonest sexually-transmitted disease in Britain: its incidence is continuing to rise.

Clinical features

Males: acute urethritis with urethral discharge, frequency, dysuria: there may be cystitis, epididymitis and prostatitis—or proctatitis in homosexual males. Reiter's syndrome (a triad of urethritis, arthritis and conjunctivitis) is seen in a small proportion (less than 1%) of cases.

Females: infection commonly involves the cervix. Usually symptomless but sometimes accompanied by mild vaginitis with discharge. *Chlam. trachomatis* can cause salpingitis and probably plays a role in some cases of pelvic inflammatory disease.

Treatment: Tetracycline, erythromycin.

2. Ocular infection

Chlam. trachomatis causes three types of eye infection:
 (i) Neonatal ophthalmia
 (ii) Inclusion conjunctivitis
 (iii) Trachoma
Neonatal ophthalmia and inclusion conjunctivitis are seen in countries with temperate climate like Britain: trachoma is a disease of tropical countries and is due to different serotypes.

(i) *Neonatal ophthalmia* (also called inclusion blennorrhoea).
Seen in babies born to mothers with cervicitis as a result of
contamination acquired during passage through the infected
birth canal.
Clinically: a mucopurulent conjunctivitis appearing 1–2
weeks after birth.
Treatment: oral erythromycin.

(ii) *Inclusion conjunctivitis*
A disease mainly of children but sometimes of adults also.
Probably acquired by indirect contact from genital infection: outbreaks have been reported amongst children at
swimming baths (swimming pool conjunctivitis).
Clinically: a follicular conjunctivitis with mucopurulent
discharge: chlamydial eye infection sometimes results in
punctate keratitis in which there is corneal involvement.
Treatment: oral tetracycline, erythromycin

(iii) *Trachoma*
A major cause of blindness in the world and a scourge of
tropical countries: a tragic disease—as it responds well to
treatment: spread is from case to case by contact, contaminated fomites and flies.
Clinically: a severe follicular conjunctivits with pannus (i.e.
invasion of the cornea by blood vessels): corneal scarring
which results in blindness is a common sequel.
Treatment: topical or oral tetracycline.

3. **Pneumonia**
A recently recognised complication of chlamydial infection in
neonates. Although conjunctivitis is a more common manifestation, pneumonia is seen in about a fifth of infected infants.
Clinically: often preceded by upper respiratory tract symptoms:
the pneumonia is relatively mild with dry spasmodic cough and
rapid breathing: the infants are not usually febrile. Chest X-rays
show diffuse infiltration of the lungs.
Treatment: erythromycin.

4. **Lymphogranuloma venereum**
A disease which is common in tropical countries but almost
unknown in temperate climates. Cases in Britain are rare and
the infection has almost invariably been acquired abroad: the
disease is generally sexually-transmitted.
Clinical features: in males, the primary lesion is a painless ulcer
on the penis which is often unnoticed. The disease then takes
the form of the inguinal syndrome in which there is painful

enlargement of the inguinal and femoral lymph nodes which later may suppurate to form buboes. The *genito-anorectal syndrome* is the most common disease in women: infection involves the vagina and cervix—usually without symptoms—but the infection can then spread via the lymphatics to the rectum causing proctitis with bleeding and purulent discharge from the anus.

Treatment: Sulphonamides or tetracycline.

Diagnosis

Isolation

Specimens: genital or eye swabs; sputum.

Culture: in McCoy cells treated with cycloheximide (or idoxuridine) to prevent cell division: HeLa 229 cells can also be used.

Observe: for typical intracytoplasmic inclusions by modified Giemsa stain or immunofluorescence with monoclonal antibody.

Direct demonstration

Specimens: smears from lesions.

Examine: for specific immunofluorescence of the typical intracytoplasmic inclusions—preferably with monoclonal antibody.

Serology (less useful)

1. *Immunofluorescence tests* are type-specific so that sera must be tested against the appropriate range of serotypes (i.e. D, E, F, G, H, I, J, K for most chlamydial infections in Britain).
   IgM tests for the presence of IgM antibody can be used as an indicator of recent infection: detected by type-specific immunofluorescent test.
2. *Complement fixation tests*: less sensitive than immunofluorescent tests. Chlamydiae share a common group complement fixing antigen so that it is only necessary to use one strain as antigen.

CHLAMYDIA PSITTACI

Chlam. psittaci infects a wide variety of animals. The most dangerous from the point of view of human infection are chlamydial infections in birds. Infected birds often, but not always, show signs of disease and this is known as *ornithosis*. When the birds belong to the psittacine family (e.g. budgerigars and parrots) the disease is known as *psittacosis*. The human disease is also called psittacosis—even if it has been acquired from non-psittacine birds: the majority of human cases are, in fact, acquired from pet budgerigars or parrots.

In Britain, psittacosis is a rare disease although the incidence has risen sharply over the past two years. Outbreaks of infection involving veterinary surgeons and workers in processing plants have been traced to infected flocks of ducks.

Psittacosis

Clinically: Psittacosis most often takes the form of a *primary atypical pneumonia*: the patients have fever, cough and dyspnoea with extensive opacities in the lung fields on chest X-ray. Males are affected more often than females. The disease ranges in severity from a mild influenza-like illness to a severe disease with generalised toxaemic features. Psitticosis is sometimes fatal although the case fatality rate is low (probably less than 1%). Rarely, psittacosis may cause infective endocarditis, as well as myocarditis and pericarditis: renal involvement and disseminated intravascular coagulation are occasional complications.

Treatment: tetracycline

Diagnosis:

Serology

Complement fixation test—for rising titre against the chlamydial common group antigen.
Immunofluorescence.

18

Rickettsial diseases

Rickettsiae are not viruses—in fact they are like bacteria in their properties. Traditionally, like chlamydiae, they are diagnosed in virus laboratories.

The most notorious rickettsial disease is typhus—an epidemic scourge of poverty, malnutrition (e.g. the German concentration camps of the Second World War) and of armies in the field. Typhus played a major part in the disintegration of Napoleon's army in the retreat from Moscow.

There are two kinds of rickettsiae:
1. Rickettsiae
2. Coxiellae.

The main difference between them is that coxiellae are resistant to drying.

RICKETTSIAE

Rickettsial diseases are world-wide in distribution but are not found in Britain. The main diseases are listed in Table 18.1.

Clinical features

Acute febrile illness with rash: the rash is usually maculopapular, occasionally vesicular. Rickettsial infections are generally severe diseases: haemorrhagic complications and lymphadenopathy are common.

Fatality rate: is often high in untreated cases (e.g. up to 20% with certain rickettsiae): with antibiotic treatment, the mortality is low.

Recurrent infection (Brill-Zinsser disease) is seen with classical typhus: recrudences may be years after the primary illness and are usually mild.

Treatment: tetracycline or chloramphenicol.

Vectors: rickettsiae are transmitted to man via infected arthropods, e.g. ticks, lice, and fleas. There is no human case-to-case transmission. Arthropods infect man by biting or by contamination of skin scratches with infected faeces (e.g. in typhus and murine typhus).

Reservoirs: usually small animals, e.g. rodents, sometimes the vectors themselves (Table 18.1).

Proteus: rickettsiae share O antigens with certain *Proteus* species. Rickettsial disease can be diagnosed by detecting raised antibody titres in agglutination tests with appropriate *Proteus* strains: known as the Weil-Felix reaction (Table 18.1).

Bacteriology

1. Large (relative to viruses) coccobacilli approximately 300 nm in diameter
2. Can be seen by light microscope with Giemsa or Macchiavello's stain, the organisms staining purplish and red respectively
3. Contain both DNA and RNA (unlike viruses)
4. Replicate intracellularly but by binary fission: best isolated in guinea pigs or mice
5. Rapidly killed by drying
6. Sensitive to chloramphenicol and tetracycline.

Diagnosis

Serology

1. *Complement fixation test*
2. *Weil-Felix reaction*   Detects group-specific antibody
3. *Immunofluorescence*
4. *Toxin neutralization*: detection of antibody by testing for the protective effect of patient's serum on a lethal dose of rickettsiae inoculated into mice: a highly specific test that can identify the species of rickettsiae causing infection.

Table 18.1 Rickettsial diseases

	Typhus group		Spotted fever group	Tsutsugamushi group
	Typhus	Murine typhus	Rocky Mountain fever; other tickborne fevers	Scrub typhus (tsutsugamushi fever)
Geographical distribution	America, Balkans, East Europe, Asia, Africa	World-wide	World-wide	Far East
Causal organism	*R. prowazeki*	*R. typhi*	*R. rickettsi*	*R. tsutsugamushi*
Vector	Louse	Flea	Tick	Mite
Reservoir	Man, flying squirrels (USA)	Rats	Ticks, sometimes rodents	Mites, possibly wild rodents
Weil-Felix reaction				
Proteus OX:19	+	+	+*	−
Proteus OX:K	−	−	−	+
Proteus OX:2	−	−	+	−

*Variable.

Isolation

Scrub typhus: can be diagnosed by isolation of *R. tsutsugamushi* in mice.

Control

Vaccines are available for typhus and Rocky Mountain Spotted Fever. Control of vectors can cut short an epidemic.

Q FEVER

Coxiella burneti is distributed world-wide—including Britain. It is common in domestic animals and causes Q or 'query' fever. Although a sporadic disease in Britain, it was first described as an outbreak of respiratory disease amongst meat workers in Queensland, Australia.

Clinical features

Signs and symptoms: classically those of a pyrexia of unknown origin (PUO): headache (a prominent symptom) with fever, generalized aches and anorexia; the pulse is slow and a proportion of cases have enlargement of the liver with abnormal liver function tests; more rarely, there may be splenomegaly; Q fever is a generalized septicaemic infection.

Pneumonia: about half of the patients have the signs and symptoms of primary atypical pneumonia with patchy consolidation of the lungs on chest X-ray.

Duration: about 2 weeks but the course is sometimes prolonged for 4 or more weeks especially in patients over 40 years old.

Prognosis: is good and complete recovery is usual.

Infective endocarditis: rarely Q fever may be followed by chronic infection with involvement of the heart valves and formation of vegetations. The signs and symptoms are similar to those of bacterial infective endocarditis i.e. fever, finger clubbing, anaemia, heart murmurs and splenomegaly. Liver enlargement is common; the disease is seen in patients in whom the heart valves are damaged by rheumatic heart disease or congenital malformation; unlike Q fever, the prognosis in Q fever endocarditis is poor.

Treatment

Q fever can be successfully treated with tetracycline or chloramphenicol.

Endocarditis: requires long-term treatment with tetracycline; this tends to suppress rather than eradicate the organism and careful follow-up is necessary; replacement of the diseased heart valves by valve prostheses may be life-saving if there is severe cardiac failure. Even with long-term antibiotic therapy there is a relatively high mortality rate although, recently, there have been encouraging reports of long-term survival in several cases of the disease.

Epidemiology

Animal reservoirs: infection is endemic in domestic sheep and cattle; ticks can also be infected and may play a role in spreading *Cox. burneti* amongst animals, although generally this is via inhalation or ingestion of infected dust, straw, pasture etc.

Geographical distribution: the disease is world-wide.

Route of human infection: mainly by handling infected animals or by inhalation of contaminated dust; placentas of infected animals are heavily contaminated; infection may also be spread by drinking unpasteurized contaminated milk from infected cows, although this seems to be an unusual route.

Occupational hazard: workers who handle animals have an increased risk of Q fever but, even in them, the disease is relatively rare.

Sex incidence: the majority of patients are male—probably reflecting the occupational hazard.

Seasonal incidence: Q fever is more common in spring and the early summer months.

Bacteriology

Cox. burneti is similar to the rickettsiae in its properties but differs in being resistant to drying; it can be cultivated in the yolk sac of the chick embryo and infects laboratory animals e.g. guinea pigs.

Diagnosis

Serology

Complement fixation test: with two different preparation of *Cox. burneti* as antigens:
1. *Phase 1 antigen*: freshly isolated strains of *Cox. burneti* give no reaction with sera of acute cases but react well with sera from patients with long-standing chronic infection (i.e. endocarditis).
2. *Phase 2 antigen*: strains of *Cox. burneti* after repeated passage in or adaptation to eggs, react well with sera of acute cases as well as sera from long-standing infections.

Acute Q fever

Serology: complement fixation test with phase 2 antigen.

Q fever endocarditis

Serology: complement fixation test with both phase 1 and phase 2 antigens: patients have high—usually very high—titres of antibodies to both antigens.

Direct demonstration of *Cox. burneti* in smears of vegetations on heart valves (taken at post-mortem) and stained with Macchiavello's stain: *Cox. burneti* is detected as minute red cocco-bacilli.

Isolation: *by inoculation of guinea pigs* with material from valvular vegetations and spleen: after an interval the guinea pig sera are tested for antibodies to *Cox. burneti* by complement fixation test.

19

Mycoplasma

There are three genera of mycoplasma
1. Mycoplasma
2. Ureoplasma
3. Acholeplasma

Mycoplasma can grow on inanimate bacteriological media. They are in fact bacteria which lack the peptidoglycan cell wall characteristic of bacteria.

The most important human pathogen in the group is *Mycoplasma pneumoniae*. Because it causes a disease long regarded as 'virus pneumonia', it is traditionally handled in virus laboratories.

MYCOPLASMA PNEUMONIAE

Clinical features

Respiratory infections

M. pneumoniae is primarily a respiratory pathogen. Although many, probably most, of the infections it causes are mild or even symptomless, it is an important cause of lower respiratory disease.

1. *Primary atypical pneumonia*: Formerly known as 'virus pneumonia', with symptoms of fever, hacking non-productive cough and often a severe headache: marked weakness and tiredness are common. On X-ray, there is patchy consolidation of the lungs. On average the disease lasts for about ten days but in a proportion of cases symptoms persist for considerably longer. Primary atypical pneumonia is also caused—but more rarely—by *Coxiella burneti* and *Chlamydia psittaci*.)

2. *Other respiratory diseases*: *M. pneumoniae* also causes febrile bronchitis, and sometimes tracheitis. Upper respiratory infection such as pharyngitis, coryza and otitis media (bullous myringitis

—and symptomless infection—are also common: most are not diagnosed in the laboratory.

Non-respiratory diseases

1. *Muco-cutaneous eruptions*: *M. pneumoniae* also causes various types of rash—erythematous, maculopapular or vesicular. In a proportion of cases this is associated with conjunctival and mouth ulceration—the Stevens-Johnson syndrome.

2. *Neurological*: Signs of CNS involvement are not uncommon in *M. pneumoniae* infection. These most often take the form of meningism, aseptic meningitis or meningo-encephalitis but cerebellar syndromes, transverse myelitis and nerve palsies have been reported.

3. *Haematological*: Haemolytic anaemia sometimes complicates severe *M. pneumoniae* infection. This is probably due to the development of 'cold agglutinins'—a diagnostic feature of the disease (see below).

Epidemiology

M. pneumoniae infections are endemic in the community but approximately every four years there is an extensive epidemic (doubtless reflecting waning herd immunity after the previous outbreak). The last epidemic in Britain was in 1978–79.

Season: *M. pneumoniae* is a winter pathogen.

Age: most patients are children or young adults: infection in the middle-aged or elderly is rare.

Diagnosis

Serology

Three tests are used:
1. *Complement fixation test* for demonstration of rising titre or—more often—stationary high titres (i.e. 256 or over).
2. *Immunofluorescence* to demonstrate specific IgM.
3. *Cold agglutinins*: patients commonly develop a haemagglutinin

for human group O erythrocytes which acts at 4°C. This interesting antibody seems to be produced as a result of antigenic sharing between *M. pneumoniae* and an antigen—possibly I—of human erythrocytes.

Treatment

Tetracycline; erythromycin in children.

OTHER MYCOPLASMA

Various mycoplasma species inhabit human hosts as commensals:
M. hominis—genital tract
M. orole—mouth
M. salivarius—mouth
Pathogenicity doubtful: *M. hominis* may be an occasional cause of salpingitis (infection of the Fallopian tubes)

Ureoplasma

Sometimes known as T (or tiny) strain mycoplasmas. *Ureoplasma ureolyticum* is a commensal of the human genital tract. There is evidence that they may cause some cases of non-gonococcal urethritis.

Acholeplasma

There are seven species within this genus: none are human pathogens.

RECOMMENDED READING

Belshe R B (ed) 1984, Textbook of human virology. PSG Publishing, Littleton, Mass, USA
Brown F, Wilson G 1984 Topley and Wilson's principles of bacteriology, virology and immunity, 7th edn. Vol 4, Virology. Arnold, London

Index